COPING WITH CHILDHOOD CANCER: Where Do We Go From Here?

DAVID W. ADAMS, M.S.W.
ELEANOR J. DEVEAU, B.Sc.N.

Revised Edition

Illustrated by Wesley W. Bates
Foreword by Dr. Alvin Zipursky

Kinbridge Publications, Hamilton, Ontario, Canada.

To all of the Families and Children with cancer who struggled and learned to live each day to the fullest and were so much a part of our lives.

First published in 1984 in the United States of America by Reston Publishing Co., Inc., A Prentice-Hall Co., Reston, Virginia.

Revised edition published in 1988 in Canada by Kinbridge Publications, P.O. Box 5035, Station E, Hamilton, Ontario, L8S 4K9.

Copyright © D. W. Adams & E. J. Deveau, 1988.

Canadian Cataloguing in Publication Data

Adams, David W., 1942–
    Coping with childhood cancer

Rev. ed.
Bibliography: p.
Includes index.
ISBN 0-9693233-0-1

1. Tumors in children – Psychological aspects.
2. Adjustment (Psychology). 3. Tumors in children – Patients – Family relationships. I. Deveau, Eleanor J. II. Title.
RC281.C4A32   1988   618.92′994′0019   C87-095226-9

Printed in Canada

CONTENTS

iii

CHAPTER 2   SPECIAL HELP FOR SINGLE PARENTS AT DIAGNOSIS   41

CHAPTER 3   EARLY REMISSION AND CONTINUING TREATMENT TOWARD REMISSION   53

CHAPTER 4   LONG-TERM SURVIVAL   91

CHAPTER 5   RELAPSE   105

CHAPTER 6   CHILDREN'S KNOWLEDGE OF DEATH   137

CHAPTER 7   IF YOUR CHILD IS DYING   153

CHAPTER 9   NEW IDEAS, NEW DIRECTIONS

APPENDICES

FOREWORD

Where Do We Go from Here? is the subtitle of this book, and a question I am asked frequently by parents of children suffering from cancer. It is asked when the disease is discovered, when toxicity develops, when relapse occurs, when therapy is stopped, or if the child dies. It may be asked at any time during the illness, but it arises especially when the course of the disease causes increased stress on the family and affects their ability to cope.

The answers to this perplexing question constitute the basis of this book. It is often of great help for parents to understand that what they and their child are experiencing has a rational explanation and is also experienced by others. Physicians who care for these children always try to forewarn the patients and their parents of the possible physical effects of the disease or its treatment. Such explanations may be helpful in dealing with pain, nausea, and other complaints of this nature, but it is more difficult to alert the families to the behavioral responses that are likely to develop in both patients and their families. David Adams and Eleanor Deveau accomplish this by clearly describing what problems can be anticipated and how they can be dealt with when they do occur. The topics listed in the Contents constitute a comprehensive guide for helping these families to cope with the multitude of problems they inevitably encounter.

But this book is more than an objective guide; it is an expression of the personal approach and philosophy of the authors, both of whom have extensive experience in the care of children suffering from cancer. Dave Adams was a social worker and Eleanor Deveau a nurse in our pediatric oncology program at McMaster University Medical Centre, where they spent long hours with patients and their families throughout their disease. During that time all of us who worked with Dave and Ellie learned from them. By developing an open, honest system of professional guidance and friendship, they provided a source of support.

Their guide affirms the importance of hope in dealing with the disease, and honesty is apparent in each of their answers. They tell families what is known and what is not known; what can be done and what cannot be done. Through their experience they have learned that each family has its own way of coping and that although individual responses may differ widely, each may be equally effective. By encouraging families to rely on their own strengths, they help them to deal with the disease. Dave Adams and Ellie Deveau convey an approach that will be of great value, not only to the families of children with cancer but also to all those involved in their care.

Alvin Zipursky, M.D.
Director, Division of Haematology/Oncology,
Hospital for Sick Children, Toronto

PREFACE

Having an L.P.* is
Mind over matter.
If you don't mind,
It don't matter.

Mark Marshall, age 8

The sentiments Mark expresses reflect the struggle parents and children face in their battle against childhood cancer. Cancer comes without warning, threatens lives, and strains every aspect of family relationships. Existing problems are increased and new ones are created. Increased anxiety, strained "nerves," financial burdens, and less time for work and fun are common examples of the difficulties families face.

This book is for you, the parents. It deals with the problems you must face and offers practical suggestions to help you manage. Just as Mark has learned to master his feelings about lumbar punctures, you and your family can learn to cope with childhood cancer.

THE OUTLOOK FOR CANCER PATIENTS IS BRIGHTER THAN EVER BEFORE

In childhood cancer today there is a climate of hope created by the medical advances that permeate medical care. For example, in acute lymphocytic or lymphoblastic leukemia, we can now expect that 6 years after diagnosis 70 percent of diagnosed children will be disease-free and, hopefully, cured.** This is a major change from the 3- to 6- month survival rate expected for the same disease in the 1950s. Similar advances have occurred in many types of solid tumors. Such progress has led to the

* Lumbar puncture.

** Clavell, L.A. et al. "Four Agent Induction and Intensive Asparaginase Therapy for Treatment of Childhood Acute Lymphoblastic Leukemia." *New England Journal of Medicine*, 1986, 315, 657–663.

continuing recognition that newly diagnosed children can expect to live longer as new advances are made in chemotherapy
and advanced medical procedures such as bone marrow transplantation are used.

BUT SOME PROBLEMS REMAIN

Although the outlook is optimistic for many children with
cancer, there are three basic problems that must be faced.

1. There are no guarantees that children will be cured. Medical
    experience suggests that the chances of cure or long-lasting
    remission are greater in some types of cancer than others,
    thus making a degree of predictability possible. In the other
    types, the outcome is more uncertain and the course of the
    disease more unpredictable. In either situation the uncertain-
    ty may remain for years. This uncertainty has been likened to
    the "Sword of Damocles" hanging over the heads of children
    and their families. Uncertainty, then, influences much family
    behavior from diagnosis on; it can cause everyone to be con-
    tinually anxious.
2. A small number of children will have emotional and/or
    physical disabilities.
3. Some children will struggle with the illness and treatment
    and will die.

When either of the latter two problems is present, the lives
of children and families change markedly and the strain is intense and lasting.

WHAT IS INCLUDED

This book is based on our experience in working with children
and families over the past decade. It brings forward the concerns
raised by families and offers examples of some of their experiences. Although it is written in a time of hope and continuing
medical progress, it also reflects the realities still existing in
childhood cancer. Therefore, we have included chapters that will
be of value if children die and families are bereaved. We have also
included special sections relating to adolescents and to single
parents. Single parents are especially taxed in managing life-

threatening illnesses, and they often tend to be isolated and lonely in their struggle with their children's cancer.

A SUGGESTION ABOUT HOW TO USE THIS BOOK

As a parent of a child with cancer, you may wish to read only the sections that relate to you and your child at any specific point in time. (Please consult the Reader's Guide following this Preface.) You may wish to read a chapter and return to it later on, or you may continually refer to it as a resource for your learning and clarification of your thinking. Many parents have suggested that they would like all of the information at hand so that they could read the "best and the worst" all at once.

You will find that this book is different from many other resources for parents. It deals with everyday issues in managing family life and, unlike many books and pamphlets on this subject, deals more with feelings than with medical information. It is meant to be honest, straightforward, and practical.

READER'S GUIDE

xvii

ACKNOWLEDGMENTS

There is no way that this work would have been possible without the continuing help we have received from the children and families in the Pediatric Hematology/Oncology Program at McMaster University Medical Centre.* Such assistance extends across a period of 11 years and has resulted in David Adams' previous book for health professionals on childhood cancer. For this book special thanks are given to John and Jessie Marshall, Doris Stewart, Valerie Green, and Jim and Penny Miller. Our gratitude also extends to the Director, physicians, nurses, child life workers, and other staff of the Pediatric Hematology/Oncology Program. As part of this program, Dr. K. R. M. Pai of the McMaster Department of Pediatrics has continually offered his advice and support, and we are deeply indebted to him for his assistance.

We would like to extend our deep gratitude to Dr. Alvin Zipursky for his advice, assistance, and wisdom. He is currently Director of Hematology and Oncology at Toronto's Hospital for Sick Children and Professor of Pediatrics, Faculty of Medicine, University of Toronto. He was previously Professor and Chairman of the McMaster University Department of Pediatrics and Director of the Hematology/Oncology Program at McMaster University Medical Centre.

Special thanks is extended to Dr. L. L. (Barrie) de Veber, Director of Hematology-Oncology at War Memorial Children's Hospital, London, Ontario for his extensive review of the manuscript. Others who are worthy of our gratitude include Dr. Naomi Rae-Grant, child psychiatrist and Clinical Director, Chedoke Child and Family Centre; Ahuva Soifer; Connie Dunnett of Volunteer Services; and our spouses, M. Anne Adams and J. Paul Deveau. Special recognition is given to Martha Jackson, Maureen Wright, and Deanna Hyland for their assistance in the typing of the manuscript.

*A division of Chedoke-McMaster Hospitals, Hamilton, Ontario, Canada.

Recognition for administrative and personal support are due to Dr. J. M. Cleghorn, Chairman of the McMaster University Department of Psychiatry and to Mr. W. R. Keddy, Administrator of McMaster University Medical Centre. Our thanks are extended to Ben Wentzell, Vice President, Reston Publishing Company (Canada), and to Barbara Lovenvirth, Laura Cleveland, and Nancy Loughin, for their continuing support in making this book a reality. We are grateful to Clare Mulholland from Glasgow, Scotland for her willingness to let us use her poetry freely within this text.

We also extend our appreciation to Dr. Mark Chesler from the Center for Research on Social Organization, University of Michigan at Ann Arbor, for the information he and his associates have provided on self-help groups.

ABOUT THE AUTHORS

David Walter Adams, M.S.W., C.S.W. David is the father of two teenage sons. He was born in Canada and began working in the health field in 1960. David is a graduate of the University of Western Ontario and Wilfrid Laurier University. For the past 17 years he has been Director of Social Work Services at McMaster University Medical Centre, Division of Chedoke-McMaster Hospitals. He has concentrated his clinical work in pediatrics and has many years of experience in counseling children and families in the pediatric cancer program. He is a Professor in the Department of Psychiatry, Faculty of Health Sciences, McMaster University. David has published two books on childhood cancer and contributed chapters to several other works. He is a Board Member of the Candlelighters Childhood Cancer Foundation, Canada and the International Work Group on Death, Dying and Bereavement. David is internationally known as a speaker and educator.

Eleanor Julia Deveau, Reg.N., B.Sc.N. Ellie is the mother of two young sons. She was born in Canada and has been involved in nursing since 1966. She is a graduate of the University of Windsor. Her major interest in public health and community nursing equipped her to participate effectively in McMaster's innovative child and family centred care in pediatric cancer. For more than six years she worked closely with the pediatric cancer team and her co-author. She acquired considerable experience in areas such as ambulatory chemotherapy, parent-child relationship difficulties, and home care of dying children. She has continued her major interest in making families and professionals knowledgeable about the social and emotional impact of childhood cancer through her co-authorship of this book and the contribution of articles and chapters to other works on related subjects. She is also a speaker and lecturer.

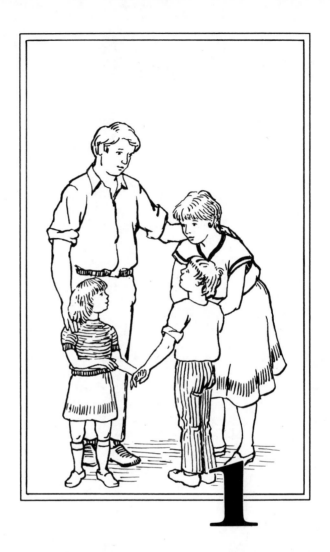

AT DIAGNOSIS

SHOCK: CONFIRMATION OF YOUR WORST FEARS

The diagnosis often comes "out of the blue"—an unwanted, unexpected, and devastating discovery. Many parents and relatives see cancer as a death sentence, and for some it takes away all feelings of hope, at least temporarily. Some parents tell us that underneath their shock lies a confirmation of their worst fears. Noticing changes in their child's behavior, a swelling or lump, or some outward signs such as pallor or a bleeding nose have made them worry about cancer or leukemia even before the actual diagnosis has been made. Other parents have been surprised at how fast the tumor has grown, and still others have been totally unaware that children could ever develop cancer. Many feel numb; they are in total shock and all they hear is the word "CANCER" or "LEUKEMIA."

When you feel numb and overwhelmed it is important to try to give yourself time to understand what is happening and not to make "snap" decisions about important matters. You will need to sort out the medical facts given by your child's doctors and distinguish between them and the stories offered by relatives, neighbors, and other well-wishers. It is common to flounder for a few days and be unable to listen or remember. This is particularly frustrating when you are trying to recall what the doctor has told you about the type of cancer that your child has, how he or she will be treated, and what drugs will be used. When you feel lost it is hard to give information to relatives or to ask for useful information from doctors and nurses. It is equally hard to think about home and the needs of other children and to remember what bill has to be paid or what child has to be transported where. Life must change, and you are probably not prepared for it at all.

3

Why Me? Why My Child?

At this time, the most common questions parents ask are "Why me?" or "Why my child?" Most of us, as parents, would rather suffer ourselves than see our children's lives threatened or have them face the misery of illness and treatment. Failure to find a reason for illness is frustrating. At present physicians cannot give specific reasons for the causes of most types of childhood cancer, so many parents begin to speculate. They wonder why God is punishing them, and some search through their memories to look for wrongdoings that might explain the reason. Some parents, along with friends and relatives, search for causes of the illness that they can understand. For example, one mother was convinced that her son developed leukemia from playing too many sports, and another was concerned that her daughter's tumor came from a blow to the abdomen. Other explanations have involved a variety of speculations such as the food the child was eating, contact with another child with cancer, exposure to weed killers, curses inflicted by evil persons, and inheritances from a wife or husband's family, especially if they are of a different race or color. The question of inheritance can be particularly upsetting as families try to force husbands or wives into taking sides against their partners. It is reasonable for parents to search for answers when information about the causes of childhood cancer is so limited.

For most parents this searching for explanations, like most behavior, is based upon past experiences with illness, death, and earlier crises. Parents want to be able to have knowledge and control over what is happening at a time when knowledge and control appear to be in the hands of doctors and hospital staff. Deep down they want to know who or what has caused the disease, how much they have been responsible for failing to protect their children, and even more important, how they can fix the blame for what is happening on themselves or on something or someone else. A review of past experiences as part of this search can either be helpful or destructive. For example, one mother remembered the pain and suffering her father had lived through prior to his death from cancer. She was convinced that she had passed on cancer to her children and that her daughter would die as well. The fear created by what had happened made her worries about the worst outcome for her daughter so strong that she was almost totally unwilling to have hope that her daughter would ever be cured. Another mother was encouraged by the fact that a friend who had the same illness as her daughter was free of disease and enjoying life eight years after diagnosis. She believed that if her friend could survive cancer her daughter could as well.

MANAGING FEELINGS

When faced with severe crises many of us tend to be hard on ourselves. We feel responsible and often become preoccupied with the future and with our own feelings. Personal emotions become stronger, and it is natural for parents at the time of diagnosis to feel sorrowful, to experience and release anger, and to want to negotiate or bargain. At times parents cry uncontrollably or become intensely anxious or angry.

Sorrow

Crying can mean a release of feelings that brings relief and a chance to think clearly again. Too often men who might benefit from "letting go" and expressing their sorrow are unable to do so because their upbringing and society have combined to make them keep a "stiff upper lip." Some fathers have told us that they must cry in private, away from their child, their spouse, and anyone else they know.

Some parents go to great lengths to hide their feelings from the sick child or other children in the family. Mothers have told us that after going to bed they cry in privacy away from their children and from people who might ask questions or criticize them. It can be questioned whether or not this is really effective. Perhaps the best reason to suspect that it isn't was given by 5-year-old Linda, whose baby sister was dying. Linda told the nurse that her mother was sad because her sister was so sick. Her mother cried a lot at night, but Linda was not really supposed to know.

At diagnosis it is hard not to be sad, and it is practically impossible to hide your sadness from your child. Children feel and see sadness, and when parents do not hide it then children can often share their own worries more openly. Even your child's simple understanding of your sadness and concern may help to provide emotional support at a time when he or she needs it most—a time when the child is confronted with anxiety and sorrow that adults show but seldom talk about.

Variations in children's responses are related to their age and maturity (see the sections in this chapter on child and adolescent behavior). Your own behavior is governed by what you think is right and what is comfortable for you and your child. From our viewpoint it is the extremes in behavior that create the most difficulty. Parents who hide all of their feelings are seldom successful, and children usually have less trust in parents who try to fool them. At the other extreme, parents who cry all of the time in front of their children convey an unrelenting feeling of doom. This prevents children from obtaining the love and reassurance that must accompany honesty.

In summary, then, as a parent of a child with cancer you will be sad and your child will know it. Hiding all of your tears may not be necessary. Time for crying alone or time to cry and communicate with your spouse may help to replenish your strength to carry on. Crying can help both men and women. Unless crying is a pattern in your own culture such intense sadness should not last for days on end but should be for short periods. The relief provided should enable you to try again to face your child, your problems, and the anxiety created by your child's cancer.

Anger

When we are uncertain and plagued with disruptions in our lives, most of us become angry. We become fed-up and we want to get rid of the problem. As a parent you probably feel the same way. When no cause can be stated for your child's illness you may wonder not only why your child is afflicted but also who is doing it to you. Blaming yourselves or others follows naturally. Anger must be directed somewhere. Those parents who direct it outward often choose to blame God.

Blaming God. When God is blamed some parents give up on their religion and become embittered toward the Church or any mention of faith. This is particularly common when children are in advanced stages of illness and parents feel robbed and cheated. In other situations we have seen parents become angry at God and try to bargain. They become extremely devout and attend church services with great regularity. When adults behave this way they have often stored up many feelings of uncertainty about their religious beliefs. Sometimes this devotion is related to a fear that if they are openly angry God will "get even" and make them pay for their anger. If they are good God may reward them with a cured child.

For other parents being angry with God is not acceptable because of intense, ingrained feelings of trust and devotion.

When fear of God is a factor, parents often direct their annoyance, bitterness, and hostility toward each other or toward the nursing staff, doctors, or other hospital employees.

Blaming Hospital Staff. Some parents do not realize how angry they are and how much their behavior spills over into their relationships with those who are caring for their children. Frequently parents will be angry with the nursing staff and will be more irritable with them than with the doctors, perhaps because they fear that the doctors have more authority and are in charge of what happens to their children. Sometimes anger also tends to be focused on minor events that may be of very limited importance. We have seen parents become hostile over the extra pillow that wasn't provided, the failure of dietary staff to prepare a certain dish, a day's delay in discharging a child, or postponement of a minor test. In many instances the concern of parents is real, but the intensity of the anger makes their behavior much stronger than would ordinarily be expected.

How Anger Can Affect Relationships. When parents become angry their frustration has often welled up to the point of bursting forth. A parent who cannot control this anger may experience some difficulty in relationships, not only with hospital staff, but with relatives, neighbors, fellow workers, and employers as well as with his or her partner. Old wounds that may date back many years in the family open up quickly when anger directs behavior. Rifts with in-laws may widen, especially when in-laws seek to blame a son-in-law or daughter-in-law for the disease or say the wrong words in a clumsy effort to comfort. In other situations parents may be unable to discuss what has happened because of their own feelings, and thus they push others away.

At work or in the neighborhood fathers tend to be the ones who may enter into verbal arguments or physical conflicts. Fortunately, actual fighting is much less common than arguments. Disputes with bosses are rare as well, but anger could lead to job loss at a time when a family cannot afford to have the added burden of unemployment.

Releasing Anger in Ways That Help. The previous examples have shown some of the ways anger can rise and surface; hopefully, they have helped you to understand what is happening to you and to your family. In addition, you may want to examine how you manage your own anger. Do you already have ways to release feelings? Some people find that physical exercise helps a great deal. Punching a bag; swimming strongly; playing tennis, squash, or baseball; or a variety of other sports are valued by some parents. Others have told us that yoga, tai-chi, or relaxation exercises have been helpful, not just to get rid of anger but to reduce anxiety as well. Some parents have found that writing, poetry, or handicrafts are worthwhile. A few mothers have suggested that, after their children have gone to school, closing all doors and windows and screaming at the top of their lungs has helped them. They said it was the easiest method for them to bring out some of the feelings that were bottled up inside. Perhaps what these mothers were saying is that getting feelings out is better than keeping them inside to fester. Ulcers, headaches, backaches, and many other physical problems can be created or made worse when feelings are kept inside.

Guilt

Problems for Mothers. One of the most common problems for mothers is their development of guilt feelings. Mothers often feel responsible, blame themselves, or turn their anger inward. They feel that they should have protected their children but have failed. The uncertainty of the cause of childhood cancer leads them to worry that they have made a serious error. Many mothers feel this way. Some have told us that they feel ashamed because they have allowed their children to develop a disease that is not acceptable to society, even for adults, let alone for children. One or two mothers have withdrawn from the world, and many have reduced their circle of friends and acquaintances.

Guilt has a tendency to gnaw away at a person, and some parents become preoccupied with blaming themselves. If uncontrolled, guilt feelings can lead to more severe problems. In some cases psychiatric illness may develop.

Ways Some Parents Respond to Guilt. In some situations guilt leads parents to change the behavior pattern of the whole family. Stopping discipline or showering gifts on a sick child at the expense of other children are common examples. Other parents have immediately instituted trips to Disney World or foreign countries—trips they could not afford—as a way of making up for their feeling of failure. The pace of seeking out faith healers or miracle cures may also be increased by parental guilt.

Recognizing Your Guilt May Help. In your situation it is important to recognize that guilt is a common and normal reaction to childhood cancer. Most parents want and need to protect their children. When they fail to do so they feel guilty, regardless of the reason. As parents we want the best for our children. We would suffer through anything ourselves rather than see them become ill, especially ill with cancer. It is the degree of guilt you feel and the way you manage it that counts.

Shortly after diagnosis a time must come for sorting out feelings. Guilt will likely be one of the most prominent. No one can say it will ever all disappear, but you can express it and control it so that it will not cripple you or lead you to behave in ways that are uncommon for you. Sometimes a person outside of the immediate family can be helpful in assisting you to examine some of your guilt feelings. Talking about them usually helps you to feel better.

THE NEED TO BE IN CONTROL

It's Not Apt to be a Mistake

At diagnosis most parents feel helpless and some, temporarily, lose hope. Often they have an underlying wish that the physician has made a mistake and that somehow their child's blood work, x-rays, or other tests have been mislabeled or mixed up with those of another child who has this dreaded disease. Although such a mistake could occur, most of the time it just hasn't happened. When they realize this parents look for other ways to regain control of at least some part of what is happening to their children.

Shock, Denial, and Confusion

Many parents, because they are in a state of shock, ask for medical information to be repeated several times. Sometimes they don't realize that they have heard it all before, and they behave as if it is totally new or different information than they had heard originally. This frequently occurs because shock prevents them from absorbing little beyond the word *cancer* or *leukemia*. Sometimes parents don't wish to hear details, and they blot them out as part of a need to deny what is happening. At other times parents don't understand medical terms or they become confused because they have misunderstood. Therefore they may need to hear clear, careful, and simple explanations repeated over a period of time.

It's All Right to Ask Again. When you are confronted with new and frightening information it is important for you to recognize that at first you may not remember very much of what the physicians have told you. You are not unlike other parents. Many doctors and nurses realize that it will be necessary to go over the same information again. Most will not think that you are stupid or ignorant, and you must not be afraid to ask for a clearer picture. Hospital staff appreciate the fact that if you understand what is happening to your child it will make their work much easier.

Will Knowledge about the Illness Help or Hinder?

Once they begin to understand what is ahead many parents look for other ways to gain control. In a positive way some help their children understand what is happening and support them emotionally. They gain as much knowledge as possible about the medical illness and, without trying to take over, seek out answers from medical staff and others who are caring for their children. Some feel that they are in control when they concentrate on blood counts or some other aspect of their children's care. Such concentration occupies their minds and focuses their attention. Unfortunately, some who lack the medical background for understanding may become upset at even minor variations in findings, and they may be worse off than if they knew very little.

On the negative side, parents will occasionally try to use their influence to control their children's treatment programs, and they enter into unnecessary conflict with hospital staff. Although this type of behavior happens only occasionally it can be destructive because it creates bad feelings between parents and staff. Sick children may sense this and respond negatively to treatment. Persons who behave this way are sometimes intelligent, well-educated professionals who feel that they can match physicians intellectually. At other times such behavior comes from those who are lost when they are placed in unusual and frightening situations that they cannot control.

Agreeing with Hospital Staff

Unfortunately, there are other areas of activity where parents can exert control and may do so negatively. For example, anxiety may lead parents to keep children at home when hospital staff have told them that they are quite capable of returning to their regular school routine. When they are desperate some parents may begin to seek out other medical experts or faith or nutrition healers. This can be very upsetting to children who are trying to get used to being in the hospital and meeting many new hospital staff members.

Naturally, those who are caring for children with cancer like parents to agree to all aspects of treatment. Such agreement or compliance makes their work easier and assures them that a child is receiving exactly what they prescribe. When you are confronted with your child's cancer, physicians, nurses, and other hospital staff will expect that you will follow medical orders. However, there is no need to feel that you are not entitled to appropriate information about your child's illness and treatment. Indeed, most medical staff these days expect that you will have questions. Many parents have found that it is easier for them to present their concerns when questions are written down. When you do have doubts it is usually wise to bring them out into the open. For example, if you are wondering whether or not your child is receiving the most up-to-date medical treatment, ask about the cancer treatment center's research programs or about its connection to other major treatment centers. Rather than taking a newly diagnosed child who is suffering from the effects of hospitalization, illness, and treatment to another center, it is wise to find out first if it is necessary.

Hospital Staff Can be Helpful

As you begin to discuss your child's treatment and ask questions you will probably develop a relationship with a small group of hospital staff. If these people are open and honest and you can learn to trust them, then you may be able to avoid the extra strain created by doubt. If you are in disagreement with their suggestions about matters such as whether your child should return to school, try to discuss your viewpoint with them. Sometimes they have knowledge that will help you examine the subject again so that together you can decide what is right for your child. They may also be able to help in another major area, the need to seek out information.

Many parents have brought magazine and newspaper articles to the clinic. These have usually discussed some new-found drug or treatment that has been lauded as a miracle cure for some type of cancer. Many such articles have come from relatives who have then pushed parents to demand such treatment locally or encouraged them to go to another country where it is supposed to be available.

Occasionally, community doctors or nurses who are unfamiliar with the current literature have unintentionally provided families with outdated or inaccurate information. At diagnosis, or at any other time for that matter, such information needs to be checked out with your child's cancer treatment specialist. At least then it can be confirmed or rejected.

When you are certain about the accuracy of such information, then you can respond to your relatives as you see fit. We have found that it is necessary at times to include well-meaning but misinformed relatives in discussions. This has always been done with the parents' permission, and in most instances they have requested that relatives be allowed to come. Some hospitals have discussion groups which consist of parents who have children with cancer and provide an opportunity to meet and discuss common concerns. If your hospital has a parents' group perhaps relatives can be included.

The Need to Control What Is Happening to Your Child and Family Is Healthy

The need to control as much as possible in your family life is common and healthy. Control through our own resources and knowledge helps most of us prevent illness created by stress. Personal medical problems develop most easily when you feel helpless and hopeless. When your child is ill you can find reassurance and comfort from the fact that you trust others and that they are giving your child the best medical care available. Your feelings of trust also help reduce your feelings of helplessness and, when appropriate, allow you to feel hopeful. No one should prevent you from learning, from questioning, and from sharing in your child's care.

Wondering About What Should Be Done

Will we put Sarah through cancer treatment only to lose her in the long run? Because many medical programs offer hope but no guarantees, parents often worry that they may be, as one parent put it, "sitting on a time bomb." Many parents feel trapped between the need to see their children treated and their anxiety that the length and quality of their children's lives may be negatively affected. Some seek out very specific statistics. What are the odds that Sarah will live? What are the chances that she will live a normal life? Will she be disfigured? Will radiotherapy leave her deformed? Will chemotherapy ruin her body or her mind?

MANAGING LIFE IN THE HOSPITAL

Should You Stay with Your Child?

As soon as children enter the hospital parents recognize that their children are in a new and frightening world. To remain in the hospital means that children will make new demands on parents for love, comfort, and reassurance. Mothers are immediately torn between staying with their sick children and attending to the needs of husband and family at home. They know that their children are ill and that irritability and fatigue make their children cling to them. They also realize that their presence will provide much-needed security. If she and her partner cooperate, it is usually true that the mother can fulfill the role of comforter and protector better than anyone else. For this reason most mothers are prepared to leave their husbands and other children to fend for themselves for a few days in favor of being with their sick children. In the short term such an arrangement makes sense. In fact most two-parent families can manage if mother and one child are away from home for a limited time. Frequently, however, the provision of sleeping arrangements for mother, allowable visiting hours, and parent privileges are set down by hospital policy. Thus, when you are in this situation it is wise for you to find out what is possible. Are you allowed to stay in the room with your child? Has the

hospital provided other facilities for parents to remain overnight? Today many hospital administrators recognize the
seriousness of the need for parents to participate in their
child's care, and have arranged that sleeping facilities be provided and that visiting hours are open-ended.

Is Hospital Care Necessary?

In the majority of cases at diagnosis physicians believe that
care in the hospital is both necessary and desirable, for there
children can be observed closely and medical tests and treatments can begin. Unless children have severe infections or the
illness is so far advanced as to cause the need for very complicated surgery or medical treatment, most physicians will try
to keep hospital stays short. Many children remain in the
hospital for a week or two, are discharged home, and return a
few days later to outpatient clinics for treatment. This treatment may include chemotherapy (anticancer medications),
given by mouth or injections, and/or radiotherapy. The latter is
frequently called *radiation treatment* and is referred to by the
public as deep x-ray therapy or cobalt therapy. The main point
here is that most children are free to return to life at home even
while they are being treated.

If You Need Housing Assistance

In special situations families are forced to travel great distances
to a cancer treatment center. Although hospital stays may be
short accommodation is needed for at least one parent and
sometimes for the child as well if outpatient care is required at the
same center. Hospital staff may help to arrange for or actually provide special accommodation. If you should find yourself in need
of help for housing you should feel free to ask the social worker,
nursing staff, or other hospital contacts about assistance with
this problem so that you can remain with your child.

Teaching Hospitals Can Be Upsetting

Most parents who come into contact with large teaching hospitals are comforted by the feeling that they are in a place where

their child will receive the best of care. Despite this many parents feel overwhelmed by the numbers of hospital staff they encounter. This includes resident and student doctors as well as nurses, student nurses, and a whole range of others who work in the hospital. Some parents become annoyed by the number of times they are required to repeat information and by the problems hospital staff seem to have in communicating with each other. Sometimes this confusion is unavoidable, and sometimes it is genuinely annoying because it could be prevented. The number of persons in contact with you and your child may be related to the fact that the hospital and its medical staff have undertaken to train persons from a variety of professions who will eventually become specialized in caring for children with cancer. There may be times, however, when you feel that it is necessary to question who actually has the responsibility for your child's care and why different answers to the same questions have been given to you by several different hospital personnel. For your own peace of mind you may wish to clarify with the doctor identified as being your child's cancer specialist, exactly to whom you should listen and direct your questions about your child's medical care.

In fairness to hospital staff it is worthwhile to point out that some parents ask a variety of staff the same question in order to try to hear the answer they want or hope to hear. When this occurs it may be very difficult for every staff member to respond in the same way. They may feel trapped and answer with generalities that are not always accurate or appropriate. Your child's cancer specialist is usually the person who can give you the most exact information.

YOUR CHILD'S NEEDS

What Should You Tell Your Child?

For many parents giving information to children with cancer is the most difficult task of all. The natural desire to protect their children from any threat to their lives sometimes changes the pattern that families have already established for communicating. At the beginning many parents associate cancer with death. Since death is seldom talked about in our society the avoidance of discussion about cancer or leukemia is often expected, especially by relatives and friends. Many parents who want to help their children to understand what is happening think about their children's needs carefully and decide to behave as they usually do. For example, if they are ordinarily open and honest with their children about such matters as sex and death they will also be open and honest about cancer.

Our experience confirms the findings of studies in the United States. These studies show that in families in which communication tends to be open and honest anyway, children over the age of 6 who are told about their cancer by parents and by hospital staff face whatever happens with less anxiety than those who are not told. Quite likely such families also talk about how they feel and offer their children warmth and security even at the saddest of times. This sharing adds to the feelings of reassurance that the sick children are not alone.

When you are in this situation several factors must be taken into account. If you tend to be protective toward your children, tend to keep secrets from them, put off giving them direct answers, or avoid discussing touchy subjects it is not easy to change. You and your children have already set down a pattern of right and wrong topics for discussion. For example, you may have already shown them that you are embarrassed by cancer or fearful of the fact that it may bring disability, pain, or death. Embarrassment and anxiety are transmitted to the children, and it becomes a topic that cannot be discussed. If you come to grips with what is happening and are able to discuss your anxieties changes in relationships with your children may still take time. Close cooperation between you and your partner may help, or you may require some outside assistance. Often the clinic social worker or consulting psychiatrist can help whole families change. Your child's doctor or clinic nurses may also be able to help you educate your child about his or her illness and what might happen.

How Children Learn About Their Illness: Age Makes a Difference

Your child's age is another factor that must be considered. Some parents think that children under the age of 5 should not be told anything except that they have a lump or that their blood is sick. At the beginning such knowledge is often sufficient. Parents can answer other questions if and when children ask them. However, when children are older they tend to hear very well indeed and quickly learn about what is wrong with them from overhearing discussions between hospital staff members and their parents. In the hospital such information may also come from other children, from laboratory technicians who check the child's name and diagnosis and inadvertently leave written information behind, or from a child's recognition that the sign "Cancer Clinic" refers to a place where radiotherapy is given to treat cancer.

Studies have shown that children who have cancer are more anxious than other children. They are anxious both because of their illness and because they sense that others are anxious toward them. People change their behavior. Many relatives and some parents bring them gifts and pamper them, and at least at first, everyone becomes overly kind. In many families discipline disappears, and as discussed later, this is also upsetting.

One writer has suggested that children learn about their illness in stages. First they learn that their illness is serious. Then they begin to identify the names and side-effects of drugs as well as the nature and purpose of treatment procedures. Later they recognize that there is a system of relapse and remission, but they do not associate these events with death. If the illness continues and they are exposed to a great deal of medical care many learn that their cancer may lead to death.

Most children quickly learn that their disease is a serious matter. However, specific knowledge of the exact diagnosis and what it means depends upon the child, the parents, and those with whom the child comes in contact. Basically, two factors are important. First, from the age of 6 on, children learn quickly that they can strive harder to keep up with other children the same age, and most want to do so. Second, they learn that they can use their illness and its advantages to control parents, friends, and social activities. Your knowledge of this possibility may help you to deal with the problem should it arise.

How Much do Children Really Know?

Many parents have believed that their children did not know that they had cancer or leukemia only to find a year or two later that the children knew all about it. Children kept their thoughts and feelings to themselves in order to protect their parents. They felt that it was easier if their parents did not have to talk about what was happening because their parents had suffered enough already. In one example Samuel, age 15, had diagnosed his own case of leukemia and shared his worry with a close friend but was reluctant to tell his parents until he became so ill that he had no choice.

On occasion parents have taken for granted that their children knew what was happening but never discussed the matter with them. Children were left to draw their own conclusions or to deny reality. Sometimes children's conclusions have been wrong.

Children may not totally understand because they don't think in the same manner as adults. For example, young children (under age 7 or 8) mix fact and fantasy together and sometimes give life to objects. They may say that the bed is bad for banging their legs or the tree roots should not have tripped them. They also use faulty reasoning and may believe that whatever happened to others in the hospital will happen to them.

Quite naturally, young children will develop their own explanation about their disease, what it does, and what purpose is served by tests and treatments. The flaws in their thinking lead them to some interesting conclusions. For instance, blood tests may drain out "bad blood" or transfusions fill up their legs when their blood is "low."

It is normal for children to try to fit information into their worlds. The only problems occur when (a) children are frightened by what they believe, and (b) parents don't help them reduce their anxiety by trying to find an explanation that they can understand.

Even older children who can reason may be wrong because they have misunderstood. Sometimes no one has bothered to tell them the truth or sometimes they haven't wished to hear it. When you suspect that your child does not understand you must determine whether or not errors in understanding are upsetting him. Sometimes your child may be upset simply because you and the rest of the family are distressed and his or her world is topsy-turvy.

These "Rules of Thumb" May Help You

From the point of diagnosis on there are several "rules of thumb" that are worth following:

1. Go slowly; do not flood your child with information. Just as you need time to adapt to what happens, so does your child.

2. Give your child a chance to ask questions. If you cannot or will not answer them, consider letting hospital staff help.

3. Convey hope to your child to help him or her carry on through the times ahead.

4. Try to be honest and to establish trust with your child so that he or she knows that you can be relied on.

5. In most situations, children respond less to information than to love and security based on comfort and trust. Whatever you tell your child should be done in an atmosphere filled with love and security.

Being Honest

We strongly support the need to be honest, but we recognize that sometimes parents need time to understand their own feelings before they are able to talk with their children. For example, Mrs. M., the mother of 7-year-old Cynthia, was upset at diagnosis because she was ashamed that she had allowed her child to become ill with leukemia. She felt guilty and could not bring herself to speak about it with anyone but her husband. About 7 months later another little girl, whom Cynthia had known in the clinic, died from the same disease. Afterwards Mrs. M. was able to talk with Cynthia about her illness and its meaning for her daughter and the family. She found she was able to discuss the other child's death, the meaning of the disease, and her hope that all would go well for Cynthia.

When children are seriously ill, might die, and are old enough to understand what is happening such discussions may have to come earlier. We believe that in the majority of situations children should be told about their illness and what it means. In fact some physicians insist on at least one information session that involves both parents and sick children. Telling children as much as they wish to know about their illness can prevent what happened to 6-year-old Brad. One day after he came home from the hospital he went out to play, only to return an hour later in tears. A playmate had come along and told him that the playmate's mother had said that Brad had leukemia and was going to die.

It is worth remembering that children will often be satisfied with just a bit of information or simple answers to their questions. As they become older the amount of information they desire will likely increase. It helps if they can feel free to ask their parents for it.

Children like their world to continue to be stable and as normal as possible. Sharing in what is happening rather than being excluded prevents them from feeling left out and therefore different from the rest of the family. Children will always take their cues from their parents. You set the guidelines for their adjustment through your own behavior. You are their model, and if you are open and honest they are more apt to be as well.

THE NEEDS OF YOUR OTHER CHILDREN

What Should You Tell Them?

Brothers and sisters usually have needs similar to those of their sick sibling. At diagnosis they are also upset by the change in their parents and want to know what is happening. Many of the same guidelines for giving information to a child with cancer are useful for other children as well. What parents tell children should be related to what they can understand. The amount of detail needed will vary with the occasion and will no doubt increase with age. Children from ages 9 or 10 years upward may be helped most by knowing not only the name of the disease but also exactly what it means for their brother or sister to have it. Such knowledge may help them to adjust their own behavior at home so that they can be helpful and caring. In the community they can feel confident in being able to answer at least some questions or understand unwelcome remarks about what will surely happen to their brother or sister.

Brothers and sisters, like the sick child, have definite expectations about how much their parents will communicate and how honest they will be. A sudden change in their parents' behavior can be upsetting at first, and if parents are used to being extremely protective it is wise for them to give information gradually. With younger children information has to be tempered by how much they can understand. In the age range of 6 to 9 or 10 years some knowledge about the illness and what may happen to their brother or sister can be equally as helpful as it is for older children. Unfortunately, knowledge does not always control behavior. Children under age 10, like all children, still need their mothers and need to feel loved and secure. There are times when they may be openly jealous or develop symptoms of some kind of illness in order to obtain additional attention. It is important for parents to recognize that this may happen and to understand that in order to cope siblings require love and security as well as knowledge.

We believe that in speaking with siblings it is wise to provide information similar to that given to their sick brother or sister. This is especially true if children are similar in age or younger, and particularly if all children in the family are under the age of 10. With children who are over 10, especially those who are in their teen years, we have found that even very protective parents tend to be more open and honest and treat them more like adults. If parents are open and totally honest age seems to make little difference, as children feel the love and trust that are offered. Teenagers and young adults will usually want to know more about what happens if the treatment fails because they are more able to think about the future than are young children, who respond to the here and now.

What Happens to Your Other Children?

At all times your other children are sensitive to your feelings and behavior. With young children especially, the upset in their lives may not be removed simply by words. Explanations do help, but they don't remove feelings of uncertainty. From the beginning children who are well are displaced. Life at home is different. Your attention is focused on the hospital and on your child there. Your sick child becomes favored and privileged, and other children feel the loss. Often Mother is at the hospital and Father, although a good pinch-hitter, comes off second best. As much as children love Dad, he may be less patient, gentle, and understanding than Mom, especially now that he is worried as well. Even the substitution of a much-loved grandmother as a suitable replacement for Mother lasts only for a short time. Movement from neighbor to neighbor or to the homes of relatives may also be acceptable, but only for a very brief period. The showering of gifts on the sick child by well-meaning relatives, neighbors, and friends adds to the discontentment of your other children. If they become sufficiently frustrated they may act up, openly display their jealousy, and choose disturbing ways to gain your attention.

Ways You Can Help Your Other Children

Most families cannot avoid disruptions. Because the sick child is a priority Mother must be with him or her. She can provide the support and understanding the child needs, and the rest of the family have to accept it. Following are several suggestions that may be helpful when you must remain at the hospital:

1. You could try to help your other children continue to see you and to visit your sick child. Relief to allow you to come home even for brief periods can be helpful. Young children especially need to see that you are all right and that you still love them. Just like your sick child they may find separation to be very upsetting and frightening. If they can visit the hospital they can see for themselves that their brother or sister is ill and that Mother is really needed there.

2. You can choose people that your children like or love to help take care of them. If they are used to going to a neighbor's home, then having them stay there when father is not around may be better than trying to transport your children several miles to the home of a relative. The availability of their own home for play in the evening or as a place to sleep is helpful. The best solution may arise when grandparents who love and accept your children can stay with them and allow them to remain in school and be at home for regular living.

3. If you are concerned that relatives or friends will shower your sick child with gifts, then you may have to be firm with them. Gifts are given for a variety of reasons. Some are given out of love and affection and recognition that games, books, and puzzles will help your sick child to pass the time. When your child has a dreaded disease people tend to be upset and feel sorry, both for your child and for your family. Sometimes when people just don't know what to say they send a present. Sometimes they feel a need to give your child the best life possible because they think that death will probably come quickly.

   As we noted earlier, when people do give your sick child a lot of gifts your other children may feel left out and angry. On occasion other children have wanted to be sick too, so that they could be treated the same way. Too much generosity can also upset your sick child. Excessive gifts can make children feel that it is good to be sick because it is like Christmas all over again. Gifts can also make sensitive children wonder whether all these presents mean that they will surely die. If you spend excessive quantities of money on gifts yourself, then you may be giving similar messages. You may, without realizing it, be saying that you too are favoring your sick child and that you expect him or her to die. It is not unreasonable to provide some items to help pass the time, but elaborate toys, stereos, and large amounts of cash usually create severe problems.

4. Your other children may be glad to help out at home. At times when life is chaotic simple tasks can help them feel useful, provide order in their lives, and allow them to show that they are very interested in continuing to be part of the family. Older children can help Dad to cook and clean and take care of younger brothers and sisters. If your children are allowed to choose their tasks they will often do so willingly and not be resentful, at least not initially.

5. If hospitalization is prolonged it may be worthwhile to have discussions with your other children to help answer specific questions and reaffirm your need for their continuing cooperation and help. Older children may appreciate the chance to relieve their mother for a few hours at the hospital and to continue their relationship with their sick brother or sister. This helps them to feel needed and to have positive feelings about caring for a person whom they love.

At times of stress families can be pulled closer together rather than being torn apart by the strains created by illness and hospitalization. It is important to recognize that even though your children may argue, bicker, and fight under usual circumstances they are frequently very close and care for one another a great deal. Secrets that parents think they have kept from their children are often shared by brothers and sisters. In fact it is often the other way around; brothers and sisters keep secrets from their parents very well indeed. You may wish to remember this when you are sharing information and concerns with your children. Together family members can love and support each other, and your children can help out, each in his own way.

GRANDPARENTS

What Should You Tell Grandparents?
How Can They Help?

The impact of childhood cancer is distressing for everyone in the family, and grandparents are no exception. Some have a difficult time coping. When they are upset you must contend with an added burden. On the other hand, if they can accept the diagnosis and be realistic they can offer the greatest support possible. If they are in good health they are often free to come and stay with your other children during your sick child's hospitalization. Grandparents provide a refreshing change for your children and offer added security by maintaining the type of daily routine that can help stabilize the whole family. They can also provide the added attention, affection, and diversion that your children need. They can offer individual love and caring for each child at a time when you just cannot manage to do so yourself.

Grandparents can also be most helpful when travel to the hospital is required, and they may assist later on when your child is discharged. They may help you personally as well. Sometimes the calmness and the life experience of your own parents lends an outside opinion or wisdom at a time when you need it most. We have often seen young couples benefit greatly when grandparents have helped out at home or cared for a child in the hospital. Their presence has given parents feelings of relief and recognition that emotional support is there whenever it is needed.

Sometimes Grandparents Are a Burden

Unfortunately, severe problems arise when grandparents cannot accept a child's illness or feel that they are responsible for it. Most frequently these problems occur right at the beginning when grandparents do not want to believe that their grandchild has cancer. You do not need this added strain at a time when you are trying to believe the diagnosis yourself and to trust your child's physicians. If grandparents go further and interfere by questioning the doctors, advising on treatment, recommending diets, and suggesting that the child should be taken to other centers, your problems can mount quickly. When such unhelpful behavior is coupled with poor physical health the strain on everyone is increased. You may be forced to change your behavior toward them and perhaps reject their help at a time when you really need it. This can be very difficult because you do not wish to hurt them.

Other problems can arise as well. For example, your parents really care about your children and they expect them to carry on the tradition of the family. Just as you do, they expect that your children will grow up and perhaps go to college or university. They definitely expect their grandchildren to live a healthy and happy life. Grandparents may feel guilty when this expectation is threatened and may have great difficulty relating to your sick child. Often guilt arises because they feel that they should have protected their family, much like you may have felt yourself. Sometimes they believe that they must have passed cancer on through the family. Sometimes their unwillingness to accept what is happening or their anxiety about contributing to the disease may force them to blame a son-in-law or daughter-in-law for causing the illness. This is particularly common when the person is of a different race, creed, or color. Showering a sick child with gifts or "spoiling" the child with added attention may occur for the same reasons.

At times we have seen parents struggle with their parents over rigid beliefs that have arisen from a different culture. Parents have had to ward off folk medicine cures, voodooism, faith healing, and a variety of other well-meaning but upsetting suggestions or treatment programs offered by grandparents. If you find that you cannot manage your relationship with your parents you may need some counseling or help from hospital staff.

FRIENDS AND NEIGHBORS

Being Outside of the Family Can Be Very Helpful

Some people choose to face their problems directly and fight them off regardless of what happens. Others run away when they find problems too frightening. As parents you have no choice because society expects that you will stick by your child and face cancer head on.

Friends and neighbors are more fortunate because they can do either. When they remain your friends and supporters they risk themselves, because they must share in the pain and the worry that you face each day. Parents have told us that there are many times when neighbors or friends have been more helpful than grandparents or relatives because they are not bound by feelings of guilt. For example, they don't have to worry that they might have passed cancer on in the family. Similarly, friends and neighbors do not fret because they feel that the sick child's parents are incapable of looking after a sick grandchild, niece, or nephew. Such freedom of thought and feeling can enable a non-family member to be more practical, to listen more clearly, and to offer emotional support that is not tied to family tradition or culture. When such help is available and those offering it are trusted not to gossip, such aid can be invaluable, especially if it is based on the reality of the moment and is free of "old wives' tales."

Unfortunately, some friends are unable to help. They are unable to face the challenge of assisting friends in such dire circumstances. Others may not know what to do or say. They wonder, "Is it better to leave the family alone?" "Will they feel that we are being 'nosy'?" "What can we say to them or to their child?"

You may have to approach your friends and neighbors directly when they pull away. As one parent said, "I had to make the first move. At work I found myself alone at first, but now it's OK and a lot of the guys are asking about our boy." Once Mr. W. showed his co-workers that he was all right and that he could talk about his son he "broke the ice." It seems strange, but human nature sometimes leads us to leave people alone at a time when they need us most.

Many of the practical jobs that family members might do can also be done by friends and neighbors. Everything from driving a family to the hospital or clinic to babysitting, picking up groceries, or providing a home-cooked meal can be very helpful when a family is struggling with an illness. Friends and neighbors can also be good listeners and may offer relief through harmless conversation over a cup of coffee. Advice about managing is less welcome. So also is the offering of a variety of negative experiences about relatives of this or that friend who fought cancer but ended up dying from it.

You alone can assess whom you should tell about your child's illness and how much information you need to give them. Friends and neighbors can be a source of willing and continuous help, and they should not be overlooked. It is hard to keep your child's illness a secret, and sometimes openness helps cut out destructive rumors and gossip. Where you live and how much you trust your neighbors and friends will be major factors in your decision about giving out information.

THE CHILD WITH CANCER

What Behaviors Can You Expect in the Hospital?

There are two considerations that arise at diagnosis. First, children have an illness that often makes them feel unwell. They are frequently sick and irritable, and beginning treatment threatens them. Treatment hurts, may make them vomit, and subjects them to strangers who do the hurting. Second, children are hospitalized. Hospitalization is threatening because hospitals are strange, dull, and unstimulating places. A child suffers from separation from the familiarity of home, family members, pets, and playmates. Admittedly hospitalization is less threatening when children become familiar with the hospital prior to admission. However, in the case of children with cancer such preparation is usually not possible. As a result it is usually the presence of parents, especially Mother, that helps children overcome some of their fears. There are specific problems that tend to be related to each age group.

Children Under Age 5

Separation Anxiety. Very young children fear separation from their mother more than anything. Children under age 3 are most severely affected, and it has been suggested that a separation of 2 weeks may take up to 5 months to resolve. It is common for children to cling to their parent or parents initially and to refuse to participate in any activities in the ward. We have found that when parents are involved in their care children's anxiety is reduced. When soothed by their mother they tend to sleep better, face treatments with less fear, and withdraw less than children who must face days and nights alone. Even when parents are present children tend to be anxious. When very upset they may ignore parents, remain silent, withdraw, and anticipate or imagine pain, especially when they think that they are going to be examined or hurt by procedures.

A child's fear increases at times when parents are tense and fearful. Fretting parents convey an intense anxiety to their child that often rises when procedures are to be carried out or when bad news is expected.

In this age range it is not uncommon for children to act out their anger or to respond as though they are blaming their parents for what has happened.

Children Regress and Behave Like Younger Children. Hospitalization is also confining and frequently blocks a child's need to be active and release energy. Young children, just like their parents, feel that they no longer have control of what is happening to them. In the face of new threats children frequently slip back into behavior expected from younger children. For example, 5-year-olds may begin to wet their pants, throw temper tantrums, or return to using baby talk. Such behavior can be reversed gradually when hospitalization is over, and although it is hard for parents to accept that this behavior is "normal" it must be expected. Children are in no way to blame, as they do not go backwards on purpose but are forced to do so as a natural way of facing the threats that hospitalization brings.

Anger and Withdrawal Are Common. Sometimes when hospitalization is prolonged we see other behavior patterns that are worth mentioning. In the face of frustration some children lash out or rebel because they feel the need to get even or to rid themselves of intense anger. Other children have become too passive. They just don't behave in their usual manner and become extremely agreeable or withdraw instead. Some children have great difficulty expressing their fear and anger and turn their feelings inward.

Problems arise when unusual behavior is prolonged. When faced with a severe illness most people need to withdraw. Rest, being alone, and being removed from the constant strain of treatment, examinations, and tests help children gain strength to face what is ahead. Physical illness adds to the need for such peace and quiet.

Children Become Sad and Depressed Too. Children may feel sad and depressed when they are overwhelmed by what has happened. Their appetite may drop off, they may mope around, become constipated, have difficulty sleeping, and cry easily. Such depression may be related to the loss of regular relationships with their friends or animals, or to feeling miserable as a result of the illness or treatment. In severe cases children may blame themselves for their illness or feel guilty. At least some periods of depression are common in children with cancer. They may be more prominent in older age groups and in children who are the sickest or have the greatest chance of dying.

Your Child's Feelings Are Probably Similar to Your Own. You have no doubt begun to realize that since your child's diagnosis your feelings have changed from moment to moment and day to day. Your child is just as apt as you are to have intense feelings of anger, sadness, and fear. Such feelings are commonly related to immediate situations, and children are usually most upset when tests and treatments are frequent or physical symptoms such as nausea and pain are strongest.

Children Ages 6 to 9

Mutilation Anxiety. Children in this age range are much like younger children. They may regress and be anxious, angry, and sad. However, the separation anxiety that is so prominent in young children tends to be overshadowed by fear about what will happen to their bodies. This anxiety is known as fear of mutilation. Since children in this age range tend to be much more aggressive and concerned about accidents and violence, hospital tests and procedures become more threatening. They are afraid that their bodies may be permanently changed or ruined or that their lives may be drained from them. Because they think in a simple cause-and-effect manner, they believe that they are being punished through their illness. They think that illness comes from having committed wrongs or having had angry thoughts toward their parents or other adults. (Later in life, this type of thinking resurfaces when parents feel that God is punishing them through their child's illness.) At ages 5 through 7 this anxiety is particularly strong, especially at times when children receive injections.

As children grow older mutilation anxiety decreases in intensity and children begin to worry that they are losing control of what is happening. Interest in changes in their bodies or their blood is common beyond age 9. It has been suggested that knowledge of such changes increases children's familiarity with what is happening and helps them to feel that they have more control.

Parents Still Count and So Does Preparation for What's Ahead. As parents of children in this age range your presence continues to be important. Even a 9-year-old boy who doesn't like anyone to know he is dependent upon his mother will give in and be glad to have her present when he is sick. As children grow older they have an ever-increasing need to know what is ahead of them. The chance to see equipment, to feel it, and to have time to get used to injections, tests, and treatments helps children with cancer come to grips with new threats to their bodies.

Denial. Most children want to be at home or in school rather than in the hospital. As a result some will make believe that they are well in hopes of returning home or in order to avoid facing the reality of their illness. Between ages 6 and 9 children

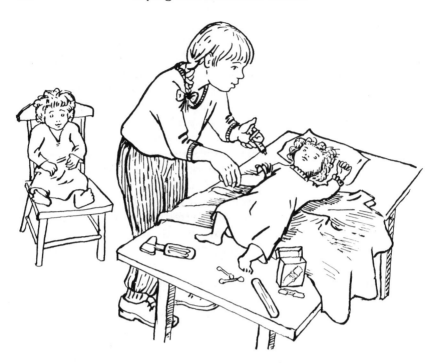

become more verbal. Therefore it is easier for parents to recognize children's need to deny and provide reassurance to help them face their illness. As children approach adolescence denial becomes more frequent. (The nature and purpose of denial in adolescence is discussed later on.)

Privacy. As children become older and more self-conscious their needs for privacy increase. Even sick children may be embarrassed by exposure of their bodies to many strangers, and sometimes you have to help others recognize your child's right to privacy. Sometimes this involves reminding hospital staff of the need to pull curtains or to close doors. Sometimes it includes restriction of the number of visitors or provision of adequate time for rest, relaxation, and play.

Play. As soon as children are old enough to play they use it to express their thoughts and feelings. Play is easier than talking and helps fear, anger, and sadness to surface quickly and harmlessly. People and situations become less threatening. For example, sick children who are frightened by injections may become much calmer after they have had a chance to play with needles and syringes. Dolls or toys may help because it is much easier to say that their teddy bear is frightened than to admit to fear themselves. Injecting a doctor or nurse doll may be the easiest way to gain satisfaction or revenge. One child sprayed water in the face of all of the medical dolls, and when asked if he was giving them needles he said "No, I'm peeing all over them."

Many modern hospitals have programs that use therapeutic play to help children. When children have difficulty facing hospitalization and treatment professional child life workers and play therapists work with them alone or in groups. If your child has considerable difficulty and is intensely anxious, angry, or sad or behaves differently than you would expect, it might be well worth inquiring whether this type of help is available.

A Child's Self-Image Is Important

Along with the problems already described children ages 6 to 9 begin to feel more self-conscious about their bodies. They begin to admire themselves as handsome, beautiful, and unique persons. This admiration becomes more pronounced in pre-adolescence and adolescence as sexual characteristics change quickly.

In this book we have chosen to examine the subject of the child's self-image and the impact of illness and treatment in the chapter entitled "Treatment and Remission." There we discuss how hair loss, weight gain, and deformity can affect children.

PRE-ADOLESCENCE AND ADOLESCENCE

Common Behavior in This Age Range

As children begin to develop the sexual characteristics of men and women they become more interested in their bodies and more preoccupied with who they are, how they appear to other people, and what they will become as adults. Rapid growth means that boys in particular become awkward. Girls worry about their womanly characteristics, and both boys and girls tend to be more preoccupied with themselves and sometimes withdraw. Some become more irritable and more apt to explode. Storming off up the stairs and slamming doors are common examples of the ways anger and frustration are released by children in this age group, especially when parents are seen to be the cause of their problems.

Friends and Enemies

Usually as children pass through the age range of 11 to 13 there is an increased tendency to struggle with both their self-image and their relationships with adults. Friends become important because they are in the same position. They are needed as sounding boards and partners in fun and mischief. Safety is found in numbers, and being like everyone else becomes impor-tant to the extreme. As parents we are natural and necessary enemies at times and comforters and security-givers at others. In order to find themselves adolescents must argue, bicker, love, and hate us, sometimes all within a few hours. Our prob-lem in the face of this type of behavior is how to help them learn and grow.

Cancer Complicates the Need for Independence

Pre-teen years are usually times when children will naturally rely more heavily on parents. They value their opinions and look to them as a source of comfort and help. As children reach the mid to late teens struggling with who they are and how they relate to others is usually stronger and more frequent. Because of their turmoil teenagers are vulnerable when facing cancer. They want to be treated as grown-ups and want to be brave and strong, but they still need times when love, support, and secur-ity can be found in their relationship with parents.

Adolescents Worry

Just as with younger children, adolescents are affected by your response to the diagnosis. You probably fear for your child's life and worry about what will happen. Your anxiety is unsettling, and you may find that it is difficult to be reassuring. Adoles-cents not only sense your anxiety but have it increased by their knowledge. Most know enough about cancer to be frightened just by hearing the word. Grandparents, relatives, and neighbors may have died from cancer, and many teens have heard about children who have died from leukemia. As a result some adolescents are bewildered, confused, and terrified, especially if they are told that survival is likely even though they believe that they will surely die.

Fear of Death and Dying

The fear of death is just one fear that adolescents with cancer must experience in their attempts to sort out the meaning of their disease. However, it should not be taken lightly. Many will naturally want to believe that death affects only older people or those who are in accidents. Nevertheless they know that everyone dies, and when an illness such as cancer strikes they think about their own deaths. Moving death down to an age when life and growing up should be their biggest concern is pretty hard to take, not just for adolescents but for everyone else too.

The Future Is Threatened

Other worries creep in. Adolescents may wonder how they will change. Will growing up and marriage be possible? Can a career be planned? Will their bodies change? What will cancer do to them? Will they become sickly and skinny? Will their doctors cut part of them away? Will the drugs that everyone is talking about make them sick? Will they hurt? Will the pain they feel now go away? Will they lose their hair?

On top of these concerns is the worry about how they will fit in. Will their friends still accept them? Will members of the opposite sex still like them? Will they go back to school soon? Can they still go camping, play baseball, or do whatever they had planned?

Loss of Place, of Control, and of Self-Esteem Are Worries

Like most of us, older children worry about their place in the community and the family. Being in the hospital is upsetting enough. It means temporary loss of place and exposure to a lot of strange and upsetting activities, machines, and unusual people. It means being away from school, friends, brothers, sisters, and pets. An adolescent's feelings of loss mount quickly when a cancerous disease is added in with hospitalization. The threat of being away for long periods now and later makes the loss of place seem as though it could become permanent. Treatments, tests, and time in bed mean loss of control, of pride, and of self-esteem. Even short periods when your teenager is no longer free to move around and capable of seeing his or her favorite people are upsetting. For the time being at least, much-desired and much-needed independence is gone.

No Symptoms, No Disease?

For many young cancer patients the time in the hospital following diagnosis is short but extremely distressing. It is a time when symptoms such as aches, pains, lumps, and petechiae (red spots on the skin) become all-important, and your son or daughter may concentrate a great deal of attention on them. When symptoms are controlled teenagers may begin to deny what has happened, not talk about it, and behave as if everything is all right now and forever. A good example of this occurred with 15-year-old Cheryl. A few days after she was diagnosed with acute lymphocytic leukemia her cancer specialist came in to tell her about her illness and treatment. After a few minutes Cheryl interrupted him to turn on the radio to hear a favorite song. After the song finished and he began again she did the same thing. It was her way of saying that she had faced enough and needed to deny what was happening for a while. You will probably find that your adolescent will be changeable, move in and out of denying, and talk about the illness only on his or her own terms. To do so allows for control, prevents overloading of information, and helps provide relief from the threat of being sick.

If Hospitalization Is Prolonged

A small number of less fortunate adolescents require prolonged hospitalization. When loss of a limb or other body part or severe pain or physical illness are added to hospitalization the strain on the whole family is tremendous. Since problems that arise at the time of relapse are similar you may wish to read the chapter entitled "Relapse," where we have chosen to discuss prolonged hospitalization and severe illness in detail.

Facts to Help Parents

Many parents consider the teen years to be the worst years that children spend at home. They do not appreciate the need for adolescents to be different and do not realize that a small generation gap is both healthy and necessary. When adolescents become ill relationships may become easier for some parents because teens rely more on them. For instance, adolescents with cancer often rely on their parents to provide honesty, love, reassurance, and security. Parents are a continuing source of strength and help when adolescents need to understand and talk about their disease. Adolescents need to know that their parents will care about them and support them regardless of what happens. Just as with young children, worries about being abandoned creep back at times of intense strain. Fears of being mutilated, disabled, and disfigured are all very prominent, and the honesty and reassurance that parents offer can be the greatest help of all.

As you try to help your adolescent remember that because you have comforted him or her since birth your teenager can show his or her weaknesses to you but to no one else. Even tears and behavior usually associated with younger children that must be hidden from friends, relatives, and hospital staff can be shown to you if and when your adolescent chooses to do so.

When sick adolescents become more dependent there is a danger that parents will become too protective and too restrictive. There is a need to balance limitations with continuing rights and privileges given when adolescents are well. In the hospital this may include opportunities to allow friends to visit, to maintain contact with the outside world, and to make choices about minor matters such as times for treatments. Allowing at least some self-direction helps to keep up morale. Making certain that brothers and sisters can visit freely can also help in this process, as they make a refreshing change from adults, are less restrictive, and keep the adolescent informed about what is happening at school and at home.

Because some parents have a negative attitude created by past conflicts they may withdraw rather than allowing times for increased dependence. This can leave adolescents feeling lonely and frightened.

No one can say that adolescents will be predictable and that the beginnings of illness will not be stormy. As a parent you may bear the brunt of anger at one time or share in the burden of sadness at another. Your emotions and patience may be heavily taxed, but no one can help more than you can, so keep trying.

MARITAL STRESS

A Child's Cancer Can Increase Marital Difficulties

We have already mentioned that when both parents work together the whole family feels secure. Unfortunately, some parents find the diagnosis to be overwhelming, and because of previous marriage problems the gap between them widens. Their marriage is threatened, and all kinds of bitter experiences are recalled and added to the strain. Such stress usually arises early in the illness.

In one situation 10-year-old Robert was diagnosed with lymphoma. His parents had struggled with financial and communication problems for several years. His father tended to be quiet and self-centered. He related better to his other children and frequently had problems understanding and disciplining Robert. When Robert was diagnosed and treated through surgery and radiation his mother drew closer to him, protected him, and related even less to her husband. She became upset, her husband felt cheated, and communication was greatly reduced. Their children changed too. Robert became more anxious and less tolerant of nausea, vomiting, and pain. Their other sons felt cheated and jealous of their mother's attention toward Robert. Their daughter, age 5, began to misbehave. She had temper tantrums, bullied other children, and tried hard to endear herself to her father. In-laws, particularly on the father's side, blamed Robert's mother for passing the illness on to their grandson. Their interference added to the existing marital stress, and the couple were already on the verge of separating when they sought help from the clinic staff.

Although this is an extreme case it does show how problems already in existence can grow rapidly. If you are faced with this situation you are subject to a great challenge. Can each of you give in when you both feel that you are right and the other partner is wrong? Can you forgive your spouse for feelings and words that he or she may not mean? Can you try a little harder to understand and care a little more?

Sometimes Professional Help Is Needed

The expectations of each parent have to be realistic. Sometimes your partner may not be able to stop drinking or may use it as a crutch, thus continuing problems that have been in existence for years. Some parents are so threatened that they cannot face the illness. As a result they change their life style so much that they hurt the whole family. When this occurs you may need professional help from clinic staff, your family doctor, or others. You may also find that you need and can gain emotional support from family, friends, neighbors, or other parents who have children with the same disease. Some families manage very well with each partner gaining support from another person. As long as the emotional needs of your children are not overlooked this may be quite acceptable to everyone. Unfortunately, this is seldom the case, as usually one parent, often the father, tends to be unable to face his child and the illness. Consequently, his relationship with his child breaks down. Again, this person may require professional assistance.

How Successful Parents Work Together

Parents who face this beginning period successfully often:

1. Give their partners sympathy and understanding rather than blame and criticism.
2. Make their sick child a priority; both parents come together to learn about the diagnosis and treatment.
3. Recognize that they must continue to share in caring and loving for their other children.
4. Share their own feelings of anger, sadness, sorrow, and hope with each other.
5. Accept the help of family, friends, and neighbors whom they love and trust.
6. Maintain loyalty to their husband or wife in the face of criticism or blame from relatives or others.

In even the most successful marriage the challenge created by childhood cancer is tremendous. The future is uncertain, and somehow parents have to find the strength to hold themselves, their marriage, and their families together. The solidity of the marital relationship at diagnosis is the corner-stone for shaping the future.

IN CLOSING

As we draw this chapter to a close there are three areas that must be discussed. These are described in the following paragraphs.

Will I Survive?

Parents wonder whether they will survive the ordeal themselves. Time after time parents wonder how they can find the strength to cope with the changes childhood cancer inflicts on their children and family. Do they really have the ability to manage all that is demanded of them without "cracking up?"

The reality is that most parents do survive without becoming mentally ill in spite of all the problems that childhood cancer brings. Many learn to cope with the strain and become more ef-fective, efficient, and caring parents and people. Many learn that they cannot do everything alone or always be a tower of strength. They recognize that help from others can provide relief and assistance at a time when it is desperately needed. Many learn that other parents in similar circumstances have "been there" and offer excellent advice and help based on solid experience.

One Day at a Time

As a parent you must find ways to help your family live one day at a time. You have to learn to pace yourself and to rank the value of activities each day. What takes priority now? Does cleaning your home to please your mother-in-law matter, or does it take second place to taking the whole family on a picnic?

When the future becomes less certain parents say that each day takes on an importance that they had never thought was possible. Most say that life can never be the same again. Many say that the change isn't all bad because they learn to ap-preciate their family more—they "take time to smell the roses."

Hope

What can help you carry on now that you must set new priorities in order to survive? Many parents say that their faith helps and that their beliefs are a comfort and a source of strength. Practically all parents say that hope with or without faith is the major force that enables them to keep caring for their child and family.

Hope for parents comes from the recognition that

1. Today in many types of cancer hope for a cure is real. It is not a figment of a parent's imagination. The length of survival is increasing, and recognition that some children are totally cured is coming closer and closer to reality.

2. An individual child is not just a statistic. A child's illness may not follow the common pattern for a specific type of cancer, and a child may survive against the odds. Although the numbers are small, there are occasions when children with predictably poor medical outcomes do get better.

3. In this rapidly changing world new drugs and treatments may be discovered and introduced rapidly enough to help children, even when the medical outlook is not favorable.

4. As one father put it when his child's prognosis was very poor, "All I have left is hope. Hope keeps me going and will keep me going to the end. I'm not ready to have it taken away from me."

Hope is a comfort, a friend, and a force that can give you the strength to face whatever comes. One mother summed it up well. She said, "I thought the power of positive thinking and maintaining hope was impossible. But it was hope that helped me carry on."

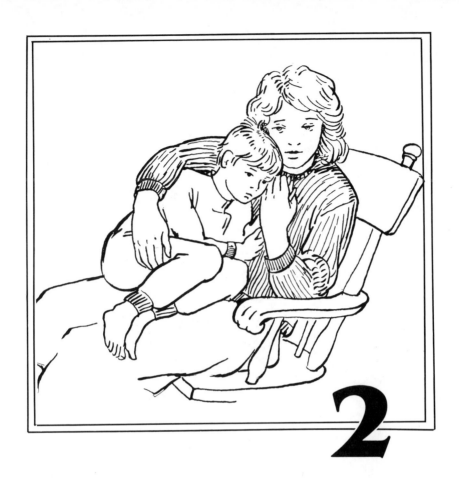

2

SPECIAL HELP FOR
SINGLE PARENTS
AT DIAGNOSIS

STRESS FOR THE SINGLE PARENT

Being Alone

The trend toward smaller families who are removed from grand-parents and other relatives has caused many parents to flounder when disaster strikes. The impact is greatest when parents are single. Recent increases in the number of separa-tions and divorces has meant that many families are in this position. The lone parent is under considerable strain when left with the responsibility of raising the children. When one child develops cancer the stress can be overwhelming. If you are a single parent with a child who has cancer or leukemia this chapter is for you. We shall begin by reviewing your major responsibilities and the impact they already have on you. We will close by offering some suggestions about how to cope.

The Harsh Reality of Responsibility

You have already inherited a great deal of responsibility. You are expected to be the bread-winner. As a provider you must manage all aspects of family finances. You have to obtain as well as spend the money. Making ends meet is often difficult, and even more difficult if you are a woman. Time out from work due to marriage and childbirth, incomplete training, and discrimination, often means that you earn less money than a man of similar age. This is hard enough on its own without the added burden of being expected to bear all of the responsibility for the care and raising of your children. You are comforter, disciplinarian, teacher, and family representative to the world outside of your home.

You must keep a sense of order and cleanliness within your own household and manage all parental tasks. You are expected to do everything regardless of how jobs were divided before and how much responsibility your partner used to assume. Even if you have come to terms with the feelings of anger toward your former partner the loss of financial and emotional support as well as the loss of sharing of responsibility for raising your children means a great deal. The challenge is tremendous! Even the best adjusted single parents find that their time and energy has limits and that relations outside of the family are much more difficult. Single mothers, in particular, have pointed out that they have difficulty sharing themselves with more than one child. They feel torn in several directions, suffer from financial and energy limitations, and personally miss out on social activities outside of the home.

Close friends, especially those of the opposite sex, can sometimes be helpful. However, without the commitment to a partnership and life together in one household the chance of maintaining every part of family life is much smaller than before. This is often true even when your previous partner was a burden. When you must face the total responsibility alone the relief at being rid of him or her is usually short-lived, especially when your child is sick.

HOW CAN YOU MEET YOUR OWN NEEDS?

When you are on your own you become the main role model for your children regardless of their sex. Your interests, values, and opinions become all-important and your behavior is incorporated into the behavior of your children. You also become the person the community sees as being the leader and representative of your family. In some ways you may be more alone than you wish to be because of distance from relatives, conflict with in-laws, and abandonment by couples who were friends when you and your partner were together. How and where can you have your needs met? Do you simply forget them for now?

A Child's Love Can Be Draining

There is no doubt that it is difficult to meet your own needs. You too need love and security, and your children cannot provide it.

Their love is valued, but it is not supporting love. It does not and cannot replace the love offered by an adult partner. A child's love is a two-way love. A child gives love freely to a parent, but requires double measures in return. This creates a continuing demand that you cannot ignore and requires a great deal of your attention and energy. The demand increases if more than one child is involved, so that your ability to give love may be strained. This is especially true as children pass through stages of development where they need your continuous reassurance.

You Cannot Overload Your Children

You may have similar problems when you want and need the security that should be part of the love found in a partnership. It is not appropriate to expect a child or even a teenager to provide financial or emotional security. It is unfair to expect them to assume more than a small number of your former partner's responsibilities. "Overloading" can be very harmful. It can force children to worry more than they should and to feel guilty when you let them know in your "weaker moments" that they just aren't matching up to adult expectations.

You Need Adult Companionship

Just as you need love and security, you also need to release good and bad feelings. You can certainly release some good nonsexual feelings with your children, but you can only show them limited amounts of your bad feelings and frustrations. Most adults need to unwind, to gripe, and to express the feelings that upset them. Because you are the key person in your single-parent family tension is more concentrated when you are upset than it would be in most two-parent families. For instance, if your family includes yourself and two children relationships can change when you are upset so that one child is unintentionally scapegoated. This can occur even more quickly when one child is ill. At times of upset children are more vulnerable and can easily make mistakes when interpreting your anger. They may feel responsible and guilty for what has happened, and your behavior toward them can help confirm such false beliefs. Somewhere, somehow you need to have an association with adults that allows you to be angry or sad or guilty.

It is also worth noting here that unless you feel you must suppress all sexual feelings you may need to find ways to express them with another adult.

In summary, then, as a single parent you carry a heavy load. You are under continuous stress to be both parents and to do everything that both parents would usually do. You need love and security from other adults in order to manage. You must also find the opportunity to express your true feelings to other adults in order to "maintain your sanity."

PROBLEMS FOR SINGLE PARENTS

When you add your child's cancer to your existing problems, then these adult outlets and emotional supports become even more important. Some single parents find that the emotional strain created by the threat to children's lives and the uncertainty of survival is overwhelming. Others manage by facing their problems head-on. The following paragraphs describe some of the problems that other single parents have experienced.

Loss of Self-Confidence

Even though many single parents have survived the crisis of separation they have had difficulty regaining good feelings about themselves. Remaining self-doubts have returned at times of stress and made them feel inadequate. At diagnosis most parents wonder how they will ever manage. They wonder whether they themselves will survive. Parents who are alone also have this natural feeling of being "doomed." When self-doubts have been added to feeling "doomed" some single parents have been extremely anxious and uncertain. This has been strongest when their children's cancers have been difficult to treat.

Intense Guilt

We explained in Chapter 1 that most parents feel responsible and want to protect their children. Some have difficulty with in-laws who blame them for allowing their grandchild, niece, or nephew to become ill. Single parents are readily blamed because everyone sees them as bearing sole responsibility. If someone must be blamed they are the only ones available. Most see themselves as prime targets for upset in-laws who need to make accusations about responsibility for a child's illness. Who could be better to blame than a former daughter-in-law or son-in-law?

Anger

Single parents often grapple with intense anger at diagnosis and at other times of crisis. They seek ways to rid themselves of these unwanted feelings and find it hard to know where to direct their anger. Like other parents, some have blamed God and the physicians, but most are apt to blame their former mate. This venting of anger toward former partners can be helpful and harmless if they are removed from the current problems. If the partner has continued to be involved with the children, however, such hostility can be very upsetting for everyone and for the sick child in particular.

When single parents have had nowhere to express their anger and they have failed in their attempts to release it toward a former partner, then problems with angry behavior toward hospital staff, their sick child, and their other children have led to a need for professional help.

Loneliness and Indecision

Single parents who are isolated and lonely become even more so when facing childhood cancer. Friendships with members of the opposite sex are tested. Just having the added burden of healthy children to raise often leads potential partners to end adult love-making relationships. The increased burden of assuming any type of shared responsibility for a child with cancer is even more threatening. Some potential partners cannot handle the emotional strain, some are too frightened, and some just cannot manage the uncertainty and disruption involved. In addition upset single parents frequently become more irritable and demanding, and their sexual drives are temporarily reduced. They become less desirable mates, and all of these factors may lead to isolation and loneliness that no one but a person in similar circumstances can appreciate.

Along with this loneliness comes the need for single parents to rely on themselves and their ability to make sensible decisions at a time when they are least capable of doing so.

Their problems in making decisions about illness and treatment are especially hard when they don't have the chance to share their thoughts and feelings with a partner and benefit from the experience.

Dependency

When lonely and uncertain many single parents have turned to their own parents for help. Although many grandparents give such assistance quite willingly there is a price to pay on both sides. Single parents say that they run the risk of becoming dependent upon grandparents again and, as one parent stated, "They treat me like I was 17. They want to know where I am going to be, who I am going to be with. . . ."

If you need your parents' help you will find that they expect you to listen and follow their advice. Other single parents complain that they feel stifled or trapped because there is an unexpressed feeling that they should stop associating with members of the opposite sex and definitely cease any sexual involvements. For grandparents there is the added emotional strain of taking on the increased responsibility that they may not be prepared to shoulder at this stage in their lives. To be needed and to help out is worthwhile and healthy, but to share intensely in their child's feelings of anger, sadness, and guilt may not be to their advantage.

Changes in Relationships with Children

Single parents who are lonely and indecisive are more apt to share responsibility with their children. This sharing depends on the ages of their children, and they may or may not involve their sick child. In most situations single parents recognize that children with a tumor or with leukemia have enough to handle and that moments shared with them should center on the child's needs and not on their own. Consequently, increased expectations are usually made upon older, healthy children.

There is no doubt that older children should assume some increased responsibility at the time when their parent has a child in the hospital. They can and should help out, but expectations must be reasonable. For example, it is not fair to expect that older children will become a parent's replacement in disciplining younger brothers and sisters or that they will share their parent's anger, sadness, guilt, and anxiety. It is also unreasonable to expect that other children will continue to perform as well in school or behave as well in the playground.

Brothers and sisters in the family will be affected, and frequently school performance declines as they become worried and preoccupied about what is happening to their family and to their sick sibling. When there is only one parent reduced attention means loneliness and insecurity. When children are overlooked they behave differently. For example, 12-year-old Albert, whose brother was very ill, was ordinarily a cooperative and helpful boy. The strain of his brother's illness and his mother's irritability and anxiety were more than he could handle. Instead of being the cooperative, helpful child his mother desperately needed, he began to act up. He was disobedient, defiant, and would sing at the top of his lungs late at night with the full knowledge that people in the adjoining apartments would hear. He knew that his mother was very upset and embarrassed. In this situation it was not that his mother was making excessive demands on Albert, but that just a slight increase in responsibility combined with his own emotional upset was enough to overload him. Overloading made him seek attention and find ways to punish his mother for what was happening.

Financial Problems Related to Medical Care

Earlier in this chapter we noted that many single parents, especially women, have financial difficulties. They either live on social assistance at a subsistence level or work steadily at lower paid jobs. They are burdened with medical bills, added costs of transportation to and from the hospital, meals there, and babysitting for other children.

There is no doubt that costs of medical treatment vary from country to country and state to state, much like the variation in allowances provided for the support of single parents. Sometimes medical costs leave families with huge bills, so it is wise to discuss these matters with the hospital accounts department and, if necessary, with social work staff at the hospital. Even in countries like Canada, where medical costs for cancer treatment are covered by provincial (state) plans, additional costs of antibiotics and other maintenance costs can be taxing. Discussion of such additional costs with hospital staff may lead to contact with groups such as the local cancer society or parent support groups who are often helpful in providing such things as transportation, wigs, and dressings.

Other Financial and Social Difficulties

Along with financial problems come difficulties in keeping jobs. Single parents must continue to care for their sick children during outpatient care as well as at diagnosis. When they accompany their children they can follow the progress of illness and treatment and provide the emotional support children require when facing medical procedures. Unfortunately, we have found that several mothers have been forced to take leaves of absence or quit their jobs in order to care for their children. This has been very upsetting, as it has meant that they have had to obtain social assistance, and those who have always been self-sufficient have found "going on welfare" upsetting.

For many, changes of job and reduced finances have affected entire families, and some parents have had to stop going to shows or theaters or restaurants. Babysitting, transportation, and admission fees have become luxuries they can no longer afford. When such outings cease a major source of relief and change has been eliminated. At a time when it is normal to feel sad and depressed as part of adjusting to childhood cancer, such change means that the monotony of having to care for a sick child goes unrelieved. Quite likely those who must start receiving social welfare assistance are affected most. Those who are receiving welfare are already restricted; their situation just grows worse and worse.

Families of single parents are prone to other problems. Children who receive less parental supervision get into more difficulty. Regular maintenance of cars and reliable travel may be disrupted. Problems of budgeting on a limited income with reduced energy and ability to concentrate on planning may lead to neglect of rent and other outstanding bills.

THOUGHTS ON HOW TO COPE

As you have read about the problems discussed here you may have become discouraged. We felt, however, that it was important to spell out the problems that parents like yourself have encountered in order to prepare you for what may lie ahead. We also believe that there are some further considerations that may be helpful. The most important of all of these is your need to avoid making "snap" decisions.

Avoiding "Snap" Decisions

If you are like most parents you need a few days to get over the shock of illness in order to plan sensibly. No matter what friends or relatives tell you, bide your time for a week and then sort out your problems with someone who can act as a sounding board. If you don't know anyone who can help you do this the social worker or nurse-practitioner in the cancer treatment program may be able to help. These professionals may be willing to assist you on a continuing basis as well. Sometimes your family doctor, minister, community social worker, or public health nurse already fulfills this role. Sometimes friends are adequate. However, hospital staff may be most helpful because of their familiarity with the problems created by the illness. Social workers may be an ideal choice because of their knowledge and skill in relating to patients and families and their ability to use community agencies to your advantage.

A Short-Term Leave of Absence from Work May Help

You may have knowledge about what is involved in treatment for your child after about a week or so. At that time you may be able to negotiate a short-term leave and then return to work later on. Often it is best to return to work at a point when a routine for outpatient visits has been established and a sitter or friend or grandparent can accompany your child for outpatient care. Much of what is possible will depend upon your child's treatment program and the number and frequency of clinic visits required.

Is Day Care Available?

In order to plan for the future it may be helpful to know whether or not there are any government-supported day care programs that will help you to care for your children. You may also want to investigate whether or not you are eligible for any additional social assistance because of changes in your child's dietary needs, travel demands, and so on. Hospital staff or local welfare agencies can often provide this information readily.

Mrs. Y. Managed and So Can You

It is important to recognize that single parents do manage, especially if they accept help when they need it most. For instance, Mrs. Y. was a 33-year-old woman with two children. Her husband left just before her 4-year-old was diagnosed with acute lymphocytic leukemia. She felt angry that he had found another woman, was uncertain of her own capabilities, felt guilty at times, and tended to blame herself. When her daughter was diagnosed her feelings of inadequacy increased. She was still upset by the separation from her husband, had not yet understood her legal rights, and was very sad. When she was told that her child had leukemia she was devastated. She had no idea that children could develop any type of cancer, and she was overwhelmed. Her parents and her in-laws wanted to be helpful, but it was hard to know how much help to accept and from whom.

Contact with the social worker and the nurse-practitioner in the pediatric cancer program led to added emotional support. These hospital staff were people outside the family who would listen and "knew the ropes." Assistance was provided through individual counseling sessions that focused upon her relationships with her husband, her relatives, and friends, and upon helping both of her children adapt to illness and treatment. Through counseling Mrs. Y. decided she needed legal help, found ways to meet travel and child care expenses, and eventually gained sufficient courage to return to work part time. She found a parents' group helpful and began to socialize again. Solid support from clinic staff and from friends and family helped her to learn to cope and to grow as a person despite her need to continue to grapple with feelings of anger, sadness, and inadequacy.

Not everyone requires the same type of help as Mrs. Y. However, single parents do seem to warrant more attention, and many staff in home care and hospital settings recognize this. Much of what is offered may depend upon your willingness to ask for help and to have a positive attitude about how you will use it.

Since your problems may continue beyond diagnosis there will be special sections at the end of several chapters in this book that will clarify your thinking and provide guidelines to help you.

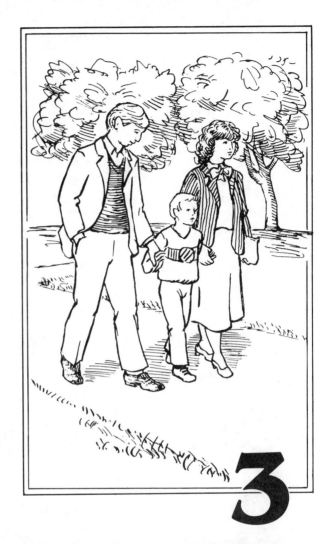

3

EARLY REMISSION AND CONTINUING TREATMENT TOWARD REMISSION

REMISSION

The Meaning of Remission

A short time after diagnosis some children will be fortunate to have their disease subside so that it enters a period known as remission. Remission for some will mean that no further treatment is required, while others must continue to take medications for many months or several years, depending on their disease. Most children who take medications by mouth do so at home and adapt well to the routine. Difficulties seldom arise unless the taking of medication is interrupted. Such interruptions usually occur when children cannot tolerate the dosage prescribed or they develop influenza, colds, or other common contagious diseases. The biggest worry is that the child's disease will return and the illness will enter a period known as relapse.

As the outlook for children with cancer has improved many parents are able to have realistic hopes that their children will remain in remission permanently. Remission in leukemia occurs when the signs and symptoms of your child's illness have disappeared and the blood and bone marrow are free, or almost completely free, of cancerous cells. For children with malignant or cancerous tumors remission is reached when the cancerous mass is totally removed or shrinks due to chemotherapy or radiation. Remission is maintained as long as the tumor does not grow back or spread to other areas of the body. Your child is considered to be cured if remission continues beyond the time specified by your child's physician.

The major medical goal during remission is to maintain it. Once achieved, remission is a time when there is hope that life at home, at school, and in the community may return to as close to normal as possible.

Life Resumes and Hope Is Real

Remission can be a happy time because treatment is not severe and many children are active, look healthy, and remain involved in regular activities. In fact, after a year or two it is sometimes difficult for both parents and children to remember that the child has been ill. The only sobering reminder may be the visits to the clinic for check-ups every 2 to 3 weeks, the need to take pills at regular times, and the occasional x-ray, diagnostic test, or medical procedure.

Remission means that the hope for cure that has arisen early in the illness can be maintained. Hope helps everyone to be optimistic and keeps anxiety to a minimum. For those whose future appears bright because the chance of recurrence is low, even the lack of guarantees is offset by the possibility of cure.

If your child's physician tells you that the incidence of recurrence is very low, remission has come early, and you have very little to worry about, you may wish to stop reading here. The remainder of this chapter may hold very little for you. You have survived the impact of the diagnosis and can now face the time that is ahead.

CONTINUING TREATMENT TOWARD REMISSION

Treatments Make Life More Complicated

For those parents whose children require continued treatment including either chemotherapy or radiation or both, contact with the cancer treatment center usually holds more difficulties. It is not that the need for more extensive treatment eliminates the hope for cure or that remissions are not going to be achieved, it may just be that the process is slower.

More extensive treatment means that life for both child and family becomes more complicated. More time must be devoted to traveling to the hospital, waiting there, and receiving whatever treatment is needed. Children will likely miss at least half days from school, and when injections and medical procedures are required the anxiety of everyone in the family rises.

The remainder of this chapter contains a description of some of the difficulties families have encountered and provides some suggestions that may be helpful for you if you find yourself in a similar situation. *It is important to remember that you may only encounter a small number of the problems.* Very few families will encounter them all.

Returning Home

Most parents find that it is a relief to bring their children home from the hospital. However, if you are like many other parents you may feel very frightened when the responsibility of caring for your sick child is returned to you. The fact that remission may be uncertain or that a tumor may not have been completely removed may mean that you have a nagging fear that the disease will return and your child will relapse. Some parents worry constantly and find that the smallest change in their children's health or behavior upsets them. Others tend to deny the seriousness of the illness, while still others recognize that they just have to live from day to day.

Most parents realize that in order to keep an even keel in the family they have to avoid being overwhelmed with worry or being unrealistically calm. As we pointed out in the first chapter, every child in the family recognizes when parents are playing games and hiding their true feelings. In some families where parents are even moderately anxious their behavior can have a negative effect on everyone else in the family. For example, you may find that you are unwilling to go out and leave your child with a sitter because you worry that he or she will suddenly become sick again. You may also worry that some tragedy will suddenly strike elsewhere in the family. You may find that you restrict your activities to the point where you feel isolated and rejected by the rest of the world. Making the adjustment back to what can be termed a "normal way of living" can be a very trying experience.

Treating Your Child "Normally"

Hospital staff often encourage you to treat your child "normally." They simply want to see that your child returns to the type of life that makes him or her happiest. As many parents have pointed out, it is almost impossible to make life exactly as it was before. There is no doubt that your child is in a situation that is far from being normal, so any return to previous routines is difficult. Children do feel the impact of what has happened to them and know that their parents, their old standbys for security, have changed.

What can help you now that you must return family life to a state that closely resembles life before your child was diagnosed? Many parents say that they have succeeded because they had hope that their children could overcome the disease. Just as at diagnosis, they found that hope offered them the strength to cope with the time ahead. When they had hope the thoughts and dreams that they treasured for their children could return. They felt that their children could actually grow up, take on a career, perhaps have children of their own, and most of all, be happy and healthy adults. The return of this optimism, even though clouded by the fear of renewed illness in the back of most of their minds, provided relief at a time when they needed it most. For you this return of hope may mean the difference between misery and feeling that you may actually be able to gain control of your life and make life at home worth living again. Naturally your response will vary with how you feel at any given point in time. The variety of feelings you may experience are dealt with later on in this chapter.

THE OUTPATIENT CLINIC

Often a child's discharge from the hospital marks the beginning of a new and lengthy association with an outpatient clinic. One parent, usually the mother, ends up spending considerable time there. Immediately prior to and during remission, visits are usually frequent, especially when chemotherapy treatments must continue or radiotherapy is given at the same time. The routine can be stressful, and often waiting periods are long and tiring.

Hospital Staff

During each visit your child will be seen by physicians, residents, nurses, and other team members. You will meet new people and encounter new frustrations. This is especially true in large centers where pediatric oncology residents rotate for short periods through cancer treatment clinics. Parents often complain that they just get to know one physician when they are subjected to another. Hopefully you will have a consistent faculty or staff physician with whom you are able to discuss progress throughout your child's illness. However, the availability of physicians varies with each hospital, and when you are faced with changes of residents you may find that it is easiest to talk to the clinic nurse, social worker, or other staff. Since they change less frequently they are often the backbones of the clinic. For some parents they prove to be less threatening and more willing to listen. They are also certain to ensure that the staff physician is aware of your needs and feelings. Most staff physicians who learn that you are upset will try to remedy the situation as soon as possible. It is important to remember, however, that in major treatment centers there will be learners present, and some will be extremely helpful. For example, many resident physicians in cancer treatment clinics are senior, experienced doctors who are worthy of your trust and understanding, especially if they are caring for your child on a continuing basis.

The Outpatient Routine

During visits it is customary to take blood tests and wait for the results to be returned to the physician. This is often necessary so that chemotherapy treatment can be tailored to your child's condition. Test results may also indicate the need for special procedures such as lumbar punctures, bone marrows, or blood transfusions.

If your child receives additional treatments during clinics you may find that the examination, blood tests, waiting for the results, and receiving chemotherapy consumes several hours. This is both time-consuming and frustrating, but if you know in advance you can plan ahead in order to allow sufficient time.

Clinic Visits Can Be Upsetting
When Treatment is Required

Unfortunately, outpatient visits may bring added pain and worry. Most children are upset by treatments and procedures, and your child is not likely to be an exception. The night prior to clinic visits children may be restless, have bad dreams, or be unable to sleep. This is especially true when they must face injections and frequent medical procedures. When young children are subjected to such painful treatment they usually cry, withdraw, or strike out at the nurses and doctors and perhaps at their parents as well. We have found that these frequent clinic visits, treatments, and injections make both parents and children anxious and are upsetting because they remind everyone of the severity of the illness. It is also hard for children to understand why medications must be given that make them feel worse when they are supposed to be getting better. Some children become extremely angry toward their parents for not protecting them from the doctors and nurses who poke and prod them, are supposed to make them better, but make them hurt a lot instead.

PHYSICAL CHANGES IN YOUR CHILD

Children undergoing active cancer treatment are faced with changes in physical appearance that accompany repeated exposure to prodding and pain. Everyone pays ever-increasing attention to their bodies and how well or how ill they look or feel. This attention can be upsetting, as adults continually remind them that they should either be better or different and that they should really be extremely concerned about what is happening. Such attention leads children to concentrate more and more on their disease and their bodies, so that some become as preoccupied as their parents with every aspect of their health.

The side effects of drugs used in chemotherapy are overwhelming. Hair loss (alopecia), weight gain, nausea, vomiting, diarrhea, constipation, weakness, and weight loss are some of the major difficulties your child may encounter, depending upon the type of medication received. A number of these medications are described in Appendix A along with the side effects of each.

Hair Loss

Hair loss and complete or incomplete baldness is often a direct result of the use of drugs such as Vincrystine, Cyclophosphamide or Adriamycin. Fortunately, this baldness is like the hair loss that follows radiation and is temporary. Nevertheless a waiting period of several months is required, and the hair may grow in different than it was before. Although there are no guarantees, new hair is often curlier and richer in color, and we have found that most parents and children have been well satisfied with the return even if they did have to wait.

Since hair is valued so greatly in society today it plays a major role in how people develop their self-image and feel about their appearance. Adolescents in particular find that it is difficult to lose their hair at a time when they are under considerable emotional stress and their self-identity is uncertain. Most worry about who they are and how they appear to others, especially to members of the opposite sex. Despite their concerns most adolescents, if prewarned, manage to cope with the loss. Many need to become angry or cry and withdraw to sort out what will happen. Once they have done this most decide that they should wear a wig, a scarf, or a hat. Some teens may respond differently. For example, after one boy was told that he would lose his hair he decided to shave it all off to avoid the frustration of watching and waiting for it to fall out.

When children are under the age of 7 or 8 parents are usually more concerned about hair loss than their children are. This varies with the value that children themselves place on their hair. Most children will mourn the loss for a short time and may become interested in combing the hair on dolls and working their feelings out in play. Even after age 7 most children tend to suffer more briefly than their parents do from such a loss. Parents have told us that they wonder how their children can play with other children, return to school, and perform other regular activities without any hair. This is particularly true with young girls who choose not to wear wigs or scarves but to go around just as they are. The problem for parents is that the public does not expect a child to be without hair, and parents feel embarrassed. For example, Mrs. M. was very upset that her son was going to be bald at the time of his First Communion, an event she valued highly. After discussing her concern with the clinic staff, she found that a wig could be purchased ahead of time and that pictures of the entire family could be taken before her son actually lost his hair.

Like Mrs. M., you know that other people will stare at your child and that other children will probably tease him or her. However, there are some points worth considering.

1. Children should be warned in advance that they will lose their hair. If they are warned they have time to prepare themselves.

2. Quite likely the decision to wear a wig as opposed to a kerchief or hat or to go bald will be your child's decision

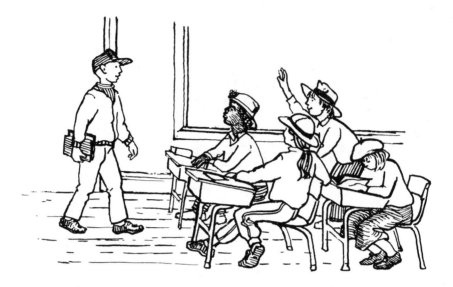

anyway. Forcing a child to wear a wig may create needless conflict and discomfort. For instance, 7-year-old Erin, with much insistence from her mother, agreed to wear her wig to school. After one day she came home from school carrying her wig. She yelled out to her mother that the children did not tease or laugh at her. The next day she went to school "bald as a billiard ball" (her mother's description), happy to be free of the wig. If your child is more casual about accepting his or her hair loss than you are, you should probably listen.

3. Most clinics have staff who can advise you about
   a. What kinds of reactions to hair loss are common for children at various ages,
   b. Where wigs can be obtained, if required, and what they usually cost,
   c. Whether financial assistance can be obtained if needed.

4. It must be stressed that hair loss is temporary. Reassurance can help both you and your child because it reminds both of you that the hair will return. Your acceptance of what will happen reassures your child.

5. No parents can completely protect or insulate their children from teasing. However, for children under the age of 8 or 9 enlisting a teacher's help can be worthwhile. Sometimes teachers can be helpful with older children too. For example, in one class after Paul, age 11, spoke to his class about his illness and treatment other children stopped teasing him. In another situation, after the teacher had explained to the

class in advance why Stephen, age 13, needed to wear a hat everyone in the class came with hats.

Some children have managed well on their own. One boy simply pulled off his wig and invited everyone to "laugh it out and get it over with," with the result that others immediately stopped teasing him.

If your child is teased home and family provide a refuge and a source of help and comfort—a fact that should never be forgotten.

Weight Gain

Weight gain is yet another problem and is directly related to the use of drugs called steroids or corticosteroids. The commonest of these drugs is called prednisone. This drug is taken daily for a period of several weeks to treat leukemia and certain tumors and then is gradually tapered off and stopped. A common side effect is that your child will gain considerable weight, so much so that clothes no longer fit properly and a new wardrobe is required. This is an expensive period for you and a trying time for your child because his or her self-image changes. This is very distressing for older children in particular, and even young children may be upset because others tease them.

When children are taking steroids it is not unusual for them to have cravings and to dislike the food that they have enjoyed before. Children often raid the refrigerator and eat constantly at all hours of the day and night. They may also want food that is not common to the household. We have seen children crave lobster, mushrooms, and dill pickles as well as a variety of other specialties. Their cravings and tremendous appetites can be extremely costly as well as frustrating, as most parents are not happy about seeing their food supplies disappear so quickly.

Weight gain may be accompanied by irritability and a tendency to cry easily. This is a time when your child will need considerable emotional support as he or she becomes as frustrated and unhappy with the experience as you do. The opportunity to discuss the problems with your child's doctor, nurse, or nutritionist may result in helpful suggestions. For example, it is probably wise to avoid salty snack foods such as potato chips and peanuts because these foods add to the body's tendency to retain fluid. Throughout the course of steroids it is worth keeping in mind that the situation is temporary and reversible. Your child will likely lose the accumulation of fluid over the following week or two once the course of steroids is completed.

Other Side Effects

Nausea, Vomiting and Diarrhea. As previously mentioned, difficulties with nausea, vomiting, diarrhea, and constipation are side effects of several drugs that may be used to treat your child and to keep him or her in remission. Although troublesome, such side effects are not usually dangerous. They may be relieved or sometimes prevented by the use of other specific medications. For example, difficulties with nausea and vomiting may be relieved if antinausea or antiemetic medication is given by mouth or intravenously (IV) before chemotherapy begins. Diarrhea and constipation may be made less severe by introducing some dietary changes along with the occasional use of medication. Any difficulties that your child is experiencing should be discussed with your child's physician so that appropriate steps can be taken to help the discomfort.

Weakness. When children are treated with chemotherapy it is not uncommon for them to feel weak and listless. They may require extra sleep and rest during the day. It is important to note how long these periods of weakness last and discuss what they mean with your child's physician.

Weight Loss. Children who vomit may often have no appetite and may experience a loss of weight. Once vomiting is controlled they usually feel better and regular eating habits gradually return. However, most mothers are quite concerned about how much their child weighs and how much they eat, and if you have concerns about this you should bring them to the attention of your child's physician.

RADIOTHERAPY

Why Radiotherapy Is Given

Radiation or deep x-ray treatment is given to eliminate all of the cancer cells. Many cancer cells in both tumors and leukemia are sensitive to radiation. In treating tumors, radiotherapy is directed at the tumor mass in an effort to shrink and eliminate it or kill any cancerous cells that remain after surgery. In leukemia, x-ray treatment is given to the head and sometimes to the spinal area in order to eliminate cancer cells that may be located there and cannot be killed off by chemotherapy alone.

Marking the Area and Giving the Treatment

If your child receives radiation treatment the area of the body that will be radiated will be outlined on the skin with colored markers. These markings must remain on the skin during the total course of radiotherapy. As a result, your child may not have tub baths or go swimming for several weeks. Radiotherapy may also cause redness and irritation of the skin in the area of the treatment. The radiotherapist, a qualified medical specialist who gives this type of radiation treatment, will be helpful in suggesting ways of relieving any discomfort your child may have.

If your child receives cranial radiation (treatment to the head) he or she will be fitted with a clear plastic face mask to be worn during the radiation treatment. The mask helps your child remain perfectly still so that the correct area of the head is radiated. The accurate fitting of this mask is extremely important, and therefore it may take several visits and considerable patience to achieve a correct fitting. This will be particularly difficult with younger children and may consume a great deal of time. Your child may also receive a very small tattoo on the scalp to mark the area of radiation. Loss of hair, weakness, nausea, and vomiting may be side effects of cranial radiation.

Some Possible Side Effects

Sometimes after 6 to 8 weeks children with leukemia who have received radiation to the head will become extremely sleepy for a day or two. This is to be expected and is related to the process the body must go through in order to return to the way it was before treatment. Children who are given other types of radiation, especially to the abdomen, may feel sick or vomit or may have bouts of diarrhea. Again, what can actually be expected can be best outlined by the radiotherapist.

During the period of time your child is receiving chemotherapy and/or radiotherapy his or her body's ability to fight off infection through the immune system is considerably reduced. If your child develops an infection chemotherapy treatments may be postponed for a brief period. This often ranges from a few days to a couple of weeks, depending on the severity of the infection and your child's white cell count. Postponement is necessary because chemotherapy further reduces the body's ability to fight infection and may make existing infections much worse. For this reason doctors usually use powerful antibiotics to fight infections so that the treatment of cancer cells may continue.

The Problem with Communicable Diseases

In leukemia and in certain other types of cancer, chicken pox or red measles may be particularly threatening to your child if he or she has not had them before. Direct exposure to communicable diseases may mean that your child will become seriously ill. Questions about diseases that may harm your child should be directed toward the nursing and medical staff who are in charge of your child's treatment. Exposure to communicable diseases should be reported quickly so that measures such as reducing or stopping the dose of oral medication can take place immediately. Certain types of injections can be given to reduce the severity of diseases such as chicken pox. Try to ensure that the correct diagnosis has been made by a doctor when your child has been exposed to chicken pox or measles. If your child has already had some of these diseases it is highly unlikely that they will develop again, even during chemotherapy.

BEHAVIOR CHANGES IN YOUR CHILD

The Strain of Treatment
Can Tax the Whole Family

Many parents report that they become more tense and fatigued as treatment continues. The strain of constant visits to the hospital and worry about their child means that they have less patience and are less willing to listen to their children. Children, too, begin to change. In the beginning chapter we noted that they have been exposed to changes created by both the reality of having cancer and the impact of being hospitalized. Children often feel responsible for having become sick and are sad about the changes that occur within the family. They frequently feel guilty when their parents are tired and tearful. After several months a combination of sorrow and guilt mixed with their fear and anger can be very distressing and may set up a vicious circle that affects all members of the family. Everyone changes, and the times of happiness and relaxation disappear so that illness becomes the major focus in daily life.

Discipline May Vanish

Most parents who have sick children think that they must devote their complete attention to them. Parents are quite prepared to accept some sadness and irritability, but when they are fatigued and feeling sorry for their sick children they may ignore behavior that is usually considered to be inappropriate.

Most children begin to feel singled out or different because they are given increasing amounts of attention. They recognize quickly that people are behaving differently toward them than they are toward their brothers or sisters. Since regular household rules have probably been removed during hospitalization it takes considerable time for life to return to normal. Consequently, when children first return home during remission or continuing treatment limitations that restrict inappropriate behavior are no longer there. Children have the freedom to act out and misbehave. This happens for two reasons: First, children have feelings that remain after hospitalization. Feelings of anger and sadness frequently come out following hospitalization rather than during it. The tendency at home is to let anger rise up and burst out toward family members. Second, when they return home children miss the structure and organization that was there before they became ill. Previous structure and guidelines for living were reassuring. Children knew their boundaries and knew exactly how much they could misbehave before being punished. Upset families and changed households mean that in order to find new boundaries and to receive reassurance that limits will be set sick children must test out their parents and other family members.

The Need for a Balance Between Overprotecting and Overindulging

Overprotecting. We know that parents usually have a strong desire to overprotect children with cancer. This happens because they are fearful that the disease will return. In many cases children do require some protection, but the amount varies just as much as parents' feelings of responsibility vary. Some parents are already restrictive and protective, and when a child becomes ill they become even more so. Problems arise when such overprotection restricts both children's freedom and development. Many children are already frustrated by the side effects of the disease and treatment. When parents add to their restrictions it is very hard for them to understand and accept such additions. Parents often have a difficult time trying to find a middle ground between setting too many limits and being overindulgent.

Overindulging. Parents who overindulge their children allow them to "get away with things." This happens when children are allowed to buy whatever they wish or are given whatever they demand. Parents who are extremely sad are very vulnerable. They want to provide privileges and possessions that will make their children happy. For some people this means having the very best clothes, transistor radios, stereos, or whatever strikes their children's fancies. Children see this softness as a great way to gain added possessions. It often gives them special status in the family and can make their brothers and sisters extremely jealous. Children who are sick may feel special, and when parents give in regularly it is easy to continue the pattern.

Children Need Consistency

A combination of overprotection and overindulgence causes considerable confusion for any child. By limiting physical activities overprotective parents have already shown that they are prepared to set limits. When parents also give in to unreasonable requests and demands for special toys and expensive possessions, children become even more confused. They wonder why they are limited so severely in one area and allowed to "get away with murder" in another. Unfortunately, when parents are so obviously lacking in consistency and change their approach toward their children's behavior so drastically, children get the message that they are indeed seriously ill. Not only are they seriously ill now, but quite likely they will continue to be. In fact, if the message is strong enough and parents are upset enough children may mistakenly believe that they are dying.

When you are faced with your child's return home you must try to achieve a balance in your behavior. You have to be fair and allow your child to live, and you have to keep in mind that your other children will be sensitive to any major display of overindulgence. Your child's physician can be helpful in assisting you to understand what is reasonable to expect of your child at any given point in the treatment program. This is particularly true in regard to physical capabilities and anticipated emotional side effects resulting from treatment. Even though your child has a life-threatening disease he or she has similar needs to those of other children of a similar age. In spite of cancer and treatment programs your child must continue to grow and develop in every way.

Difficulty with Discipline and What You Can Do About It

As noted earlier, children with cancer have to be treated as normally as possible within their own circumstances. Because they still need love, affection, and guidance they need limits set on their behavior. The pitfalls of overindulgence, overprotection, and lack of limits have already been discussed. However, the dilemma remains: How do you handle outbursts of anger and frustration at home and in the clinic? Discipline is especially difficult when you realize that your child is reacting to frustration that would be absent if cancer were not a factor. In some ways your child has every right to feel angry and helpless or trapped. Medication often adds to children's anger and irritability, and if you realize this it is even more difficult for you to provide the discipline that is needed. As we pointed out earlier, irritability, sleeplessness, and a tendency to cry easily have all been associated with the use of the drug prednisone. Other drugs may upset some children in a similar manner.

When your child is frustrated, angry, and demanding you may feel that your discipline will just add to his or her frustrations. Yet without controls it is extremely difficult to live with your child, and his or her behavior is a source of frustration for everyone concerned. Regardless of what happens, your child does need your help to set limits on behavior and to channel anger constructively. Without such attention, the child may feel that you have truly given up on him or her. How, then, do you manage angry outbursts and behavior that you cannot tolerate? There are several requirements. First, you must have some basic knowledge of what can be reasonably expected of your child given the effects of illness and treatment. It is helpful to try and remember what capabilities your child had before, how you treated the child then, and how he or she has changed.

Second, you must assess how you have changed as well. Often discussions with your partner will help you do this. Third, assessments of your child and yourself may lead you to specific plans of action. For example, you may conclude that you must change your current approach to discipline. A different approach may simply mean reintroducing the consistency that used to be in your household along with reasonable limits that all of the children in your family understand. Even if you must make minor concessions for your sick child, your other children are more apt to tolerate them when expectations are clear and the household is orderly.

When considering changes in discipline you may have to find new methods for punishment and reward. For instance, a number of parents of children with leukemia have had to stop spanking their children because they bruise easily. They have learned through experience that removing privileges is as effective as or more effective than spanking. Others have found that when a child has been angry and lashed out at brothers and sisters or other children the introduction of suitable ways to allow the child to express anger has helped solve the problem. For example, one child benefited from the use of an inflated punching bag and another pounded nails in his father's workshop. Centers, where there are summer camps for children with cancer, provide opportunities to share feelings and make new friends.*

Overcoming Social Isolation

You may find that some discipline problems arise from your child's relationship difficulties with children of his or her own age and with people who are outside of the family. If children have not been to school for a long time they tend to feel singled out and alone. Their isolation may lead them to reject or be rejected by their friends. They feel left out and fall behind in school and play. When this happens they may release their frustration by "picking on" younger children or they may be the victims when peers make fun of them because they look different or because they have had to remain at home and miss school.

When sick children are misbehaving the return to school can be helpful. The return challenges their minds and forces them to try to renew relationships outside of the family. After a while family members become stale, home is boring, and family relationships can become strained. Getting back with children their own age and seeing their teachers again can be a much-

---

* see Appendix E: Summer Camps for Children with Cancer, p. 296.

needed relief, especially if the process goes smoothly. As one writer put it, school for the child is the same as work for the adult. School is one means of returning to a more "normal" life away from hospital and clinic.

HELPING YOUR CHILD TO RETURN TO SCHOOL CAN BE A MAJOR CHALLENGE

Although school can be helpful, returning there may mean a big step. Many parents point out that going back to school has created a great deal of anxiety and apprehension for everyone. The encounter with cancer, hospitalization, and extensive treatment has meant that the total family has been removed from the school system. Children have lost contact with their classmates and have spent considerable time away from their normal studies. When this happens some fall behind while others who have had a home tutor may have been fortunate enough to keep up with their school work. Even for the most fortunate the learning process has been quite different and going back to the classroom means a major adjustment.

You are confronted with a number of concerns when you and your child must face this problem. Changes in children's physical appearance may mean that they feel that others will no longer like them or accept them. In fact, they may not like themselves. The fear of what others think and their negative feelings about themselves may mean that it is very difficult for them to adjust both physically and emotionally to school. If they have lost hair, gained or lost weight, lost a limb, or have ugly surgical scars, they may worry that they will be teased and rejected by their peers. Naturally, you will worry that other children and teachers may not be able to adjust to the changes in your child. You will likely wonder for days or weeks in advance what will happen. Frequently, resolution of your uncertainty will depend upon the amount of preparation that your child's teacher and classmates have received in advance of your child's return. A factual letter from your child's doctor to the school may help the teachers understand your child's illness.[*]

Like most parents you may feel reluctant to let your child go because you cannot protect the child in school in the same

---

[*]See Appendix C: "Additional Reading Material for Teachers."

way that you can at home. Starting school means increased risks of infection, especially during periods of chemotherapy treatment when resistance is lowered. If your child has leukemia, you may be concerned that he or she will be exposed to contagious diseases such as chicken pox and measles. You may also worry that your child might overexert himself or herself in the desire to be like friends or withdraw because he or she is frightened of rejection by teachers and classmates.

Almost every parent has the desire to protect his or her child from any physical or emotional abuse. Some have suggested that they have felt that their children had suffered enough without forcing them to go back to school. You may feel the same way, yet your child has the need to be with peers and friends and to do what he or she would normally do if the cancer hadn't developed. You may have to recognize that if you stop your child from going to school, you may block the child's need to be like brothers and sisters and friends, to be the same as everyone else, and most important of all, to have a sense of belonging. Erin, age 7, demonstrated the strength of this need and children's determination to fulfill it. She was determined to stay in school and return there for whatever time remained in the school day following each treatment for leukemia. She refused to miss anything. On treatment days she would insist on doing any work she had missed while the other children were out at recess. Her mother and teacher felt that this was Erin's way of fighting to be like everyone else. Her determination persisted,and she retained her place at the top of the class.

On the negative side, a few children may respond like 7-year-old Jane, who tried to use her illness to gain added attention and special favors. She would be too tired to complete her school work and would ask for extra assistance because she was ill. Her mother and teacher had to work together to sort out what Jane could really do and just how much she actually needed to be pampered. Her behavior spilled over into gym classes, where she would feign illness or fatigue to avoid participating.

Teachers Can Help

Treatment offers the opportunity for remission for many children and for cure for an increasing number each year. Consequently, the possibility of a long and healthy future for your child has to be taken into account so that he or she can regain as much as possible of what has been lost through illness. Because of this many parents have reported that they have helped to ease their children's reentry into the school system. A number have met with the teacher, principal, and other school personnel who are in direct contact with their children. They have found that the amount of information about cancer and the amount of guidance and support that teachers receive greatly influences their attitude toward a child's return to school.

For most teachers, contact with a child who has cancer is a new experience. It taxes their emotions, frightens them, and raises many questions about a child's capabilities. Without adequate information the teacher's attitude may be negative. One mother, for example, reported that her child's teacher told her that she could not understand the need to spend extra time with her daughter because it would be only a few months before the child would die anyway. In all fairness, all that the teacher knew at that point was that the child had leukemia. What she didn't know was that the child was in complete remission and that there was a great deal of hope that the child would be cured.

School personnel who understand your child's disease and treatment can have a realistic approach, appropriate expectations, and the same positive outlook for your child that you have. Accurate knowledge will help prevent teachers from over-protecting your child while ensuring that necessary precautions are taken to avoid contagious and communicable diseases. In addition, if your child has physical limitations some adjustments can often be made. Parents also report that meeting with teachers prior to a child's return to school enables teachers to prepare both themselves and their pupils. As we mentioned in our discussion on hair loss, class preparation can be especially helpful if your child has undergone any changes in appearance.

When parents, teacher, and principal work together many have found that support can be mutual. Just as it is difficult for you to send your child to school, it is equally difficult for the teacher to work with children who may be absent frequently and be quite different physically and emotionally than they were before the illness began. Special needs and concessions may have to be made, and parent-teacher communication helps make these realistic. The value of this parent-teacher relationship increases on a continuing basis as teachers can be helpful in monitoring your child's adjustment to school and in taking an active role if your child is mistreated by other children.

HOW CAN YOU COPE?

Values May Change

There is no question that the treatment of cancer has such a major impact on everyone in the family that personal relationships are bound to change. Parents report that the daily stress and anxiety of having a child with cancer means that each family member has to adapt to new roles and responsibilities. Everyone in the family knows that they must make adjustments in order to live with the child's illness. As one mother of a 6-year-old girl with leukemia suggested, "My husband and I came to realize that what is really important is life itself, and all other things are just incidental. To keep everyone happy is what counts." It is a tremendous challenge for family members to make such sweeping changes and to place their highest values on daily experiences with each other. This is especially true when children have illnesses that threaten their lives.

The Problem of Separate Roles

When parents must assume new or drastically changed roles within the family there is a danger that they will become locked into separate roles. Mothers who work often have to temporarily give up their employment in order to care for their child. They are the ones who come to the hospital with their children and provide the warmth, love, and support necessary to help their sons or daughters through the treatment process. Fathers, on the other hand, frequently tend to remain in the role of wage-earner. Unlike mothers—who deal with the disease on a day-to-day basis and become very familiar with the treatment procedures, blood counts, and medical routines—fathers may tend to be left out. Many fathers are not as deeply involved in the clinic visits and treatments because of the demands of their jobs. Others who are frightened or distressed by their child's illness and treatment program may use their work as an excuse not to be involved. Still others who earn wages on an hourly basis may create financial distress for the family if they allow clinic visits to prevent them from working.

As a result of the differences between the roles of mother and father a separateness can develop that makes it difficult for parents to give emotional support to each other. We have frequently seen mothers who, under the strain of seeing their child go through difficult procedures, have become extremely angry and resentful because the father is absent. They feel that their husbands are neglecting them and their sick children and are failing to see the agony and anguish that their children must face. This problem becomes greatest at times of crisis. In fact, fathers may feel very left out. They may feel that mothers are exaggerating or telling them half-truths or mixing up the information. When this happens parents feel less willing to discuss their problems with each other and ill feelings can grow rapidly.

Sharing Usually Helps

Parents may be able to understand each other more easily when they share in their child's care together. Sharing often helps them to cooperate and negotiate workable roles and responsibilities. For example, fathers can assist mothers with some of the practical problems of transporation, care of other children in the home, and management of finances. The attention and involvement of the father can help to avoid some of the problems we have seen in families where the illness has so preoccupied the mother that details of family management have been ignored. For instance, in families where the mother has controlled household finances her failure to manage the financial drain of the illness has left some families in a mess. The additional funds for transportation, extra food, medications, and items not covered by insurance (such as antibiotics, wigs, clothing, and even added costs of walkers or prostheses) have all been factors that have added to the difficulties. The attention of the father may not totally remove such problems, but his involvement may lessen the impact.

Intense Treatment Programs
Are Difficult for Everyone

When a child must face an extensive treatment program the strain of working, taking a child to the hospital, and caring for other children is intense. Even when parents do communicate and help each other the enormous demands placed on both of them mean that very little time or energy is left for talking with each other or sharing fears, anger, and frustration. For some parents sexual activity totally disappears. Distressed adults are often unable to express their feelings of love and affection for

one another, but few couples are aware of it until they experience a crisis like childhood cancer. Other parents feel that
they are on the brink of disaster and that their world will collapse further. Sometimes they feel that they are just being built
up by seeing their child improve and that in reality they are being
set up for a bigger fall, which will come when the disease returns.

The Negative Effects of Stress

Such emotional tension can strain any marriage and for some,
negative results just cannot be avoided. If marriage problems
were there before the child was diagnosed they may get worse.
Good feelings diminish and are replaced by the tendency to
blame or continually find fault with the other partner. Under
continuing strain problems with in-laws also increase. Their
unwelcome interference brings back dislikes, hatred, and
jealousies. As marital and family relationships deteriorate
everyone suffers, including the sick child and other children in
the family. Some writers have reported that there is a higher
rate of separation and divorce in couples with children who
have cancer than in the general population. Although we would
suggest that this is not necessarily the case, the fact remains
that the stress of illness added to existing family problems can
lead to separation and divorce. For instance, we have seen
parents separate because they have been unable to face what is
happening to their child. Misdirecting anger about the illness
by blaming their partner, feeling guilty about allowing their
child to become ill, and failing to trust one another have all contributed to bitter and open conflict between parents. Their
fatigue and emotional exhaustion have made it difficult for
them to think clearly and resolve disputes. When communication has deteriorated relationships have gone from bad to
worse.

Some Positive Guidelines for Coping

On the positive side, we believe that most parents can cope. We
also know that many families can and do remain together. A lot of
them already have considerable strength but may need help to
recognize it and use it. For example, you may have to learn how
to put your family's strength to work so that you and your partner can pull together rather than pull apart. Here are some
guidelines which should be helpful for you.

1. If you and your partner are *familiar with the illness and the plan for treatment*, your knowledge of what is ahead will probably help both of you. In addition to knowing why the treatment is being given you will be able to recognize the good and the bad signs of what the illness or treatment is doing to your child. You may also be reassured if you know that the treatment is the best available and that survival has increased in many types of cancer. When you know that your child is receiving excellent medical care you can feel that you have at least some degree of control in the situation. Your comfort with your own knowledge about what is happening will help you to assist your child in understanding his or her illness and to face whatever is ahead.

2. *Active involvement in the treatment* of your child can help you adapt to the illness. You can benefit from knowing that you are providing the understanding, support, and encouragement that your child needs to help diminish his or her anxiety. Your continuing relationship with your child can help to increase his or her trust in the doctors and nurses so that life is easier for everyone including yourself. When you are involved and busy you have less time to worry and you will gradually become conditioned to the impact of the illness.

3. Much has been written about the pros and cons of *denying what is happening.* Quite naturally, if your child begins to look and feel better you may think that perhaps the illness will not return. At least you may partially believe this even though at the back of your mind you know that it may not be the case. The mother of one little boy with leukemia pointed out that she moved in and out of denying. There were times when she didn't want to believe that he had the disease and other times when she found that she watched him very carefully and was very much aware of the fact that he could relapse. In reality, denial can be extremely healthy and provides the relief you may need to cope in the weeks, months, and years ahead. The clinic visits and medications that are taken at home are often the only reminders that your child is sick. Parents who cope well tell us that they "don't constantly think about the disease" and that they "live one day at a time."

   On the other hand, denial can be overplayed, and on a few occasions we have had to remind the parents that their children have been ill and require continued treatment. This has usually arisen because parents have become careless about giving their children much-needed medication. One mother pointed out to us that she was extremely resentful because we had reminded her about her daughter's cancer at a time when she wanted to forget it. This may have been a very fair point in her case. Her family life had returned to a comfortable routine and clinic visits were upsetting enough without us reminding her of the problems that might be ahead. However, we believed that she needed to be reminded to provide her child with small amounts of protection and to pay attention to the continued need to give the prescribed medication. We continue to believe that some parents may require such reminding.

In summary then, if your child's health is not jeopardized it is all right to forget about the illness—even for extended periods of time—and return to normal activities that provide relief from the stress of the disease. Just as children need to have time to deny what is happening or to work it through in their play activities, parents need time off to think about pleasant, happy, and restful times in life. Families also need opportunities for play together and for respite and relief. Moderate amounts of denial are healthy.

4. Adult cancer patients tell us that they must have *hope*; so must parents of children with cancer. Without hope it is very difficult for them to accept very aggressive treatment programs and to endure the side effects that accompany them. Parents who lose hope completely are of little help to children who really need support and encouragement during a difficult period of treatment. Without hope parents tend to overprotect and overindulge their children to the point where children feel that their parents have totally given up on them. For most children this is very frightening and upsetting, and they feel guilty. They blame themselves for hurting their parents. They also may feel rejected and worried that they have done something terrible to make their parents stop loving them.

Since your child is being treated and since the future is uncertain, it is worth noting that there are *varying degrees of hope*. In situations where your child faces a bleak prognosis (as discussed later in the section on relapse) a reduction in hope may be very realistic. However, at this point if your child is in remission or on the brink of remission there is a need to gain as much as possible from whatever hope you have. Physicians, nurses and hospital staff can help make you keep your hopes realistic. Your hope can mean that you may be able to provide the security and emotional support that your child desperately needs from the family.

5. If your Cancer Center has a parents' group, you may find it provides you with support and opportunities to share your feelings and concerns.*

SIBLINGS

What Siblings May Feel

Children with cancer are not the only ones whose lives are disrupted. Brothers and sisters must learn to adjust to a situation that has not only disturbed their family but has added many personal fears and uncertainties to their lives too. As parents you may find it extremely difficult to give added attention to your other children when your sick child is demanding so much from you. Yet brothers and sisters need help to work through a variety of feelings. They may feel jealous at the added attention that your sick child receives. If gifts and special privileges are part of being ill they may feel cheated, left out, and resentful. When some children feel jealous they also feel guilty. They feel guilty that they are actually trying to inflict other problems on you at a time when you are already overwhelmed. In some instances brothers and sisters also believe that they have caused the illness. A simple cause and effect reaction is especially common with children in the age range of 5 to 8. Even older children may feel that perhaps something they said or did caused the illness. Some children also feel bad because they are well and their brother or sister is ill.

Family Life Is Disrupted

Many problems for siblings arise when family activities are planned around the sick child at diagnosis and the pattern continues indefinitely. Regular outings and activities that brothers and sisters usually enjoy are dropped. Clinic visits, side effects of medication, and a whole host of other illness-related problems encroach upon their lives. They suffer from a real or imagined loss of hope and security. They know that your energies and attention are directed toward your sick child, and they begin to feel isolated. Isolation can lead to other problems such as difficulties in school and acting out against other children.

* see Appendix E: Parents' Groups, p. 295.

Brothers and sisters are put in a very difficult position when they are upset and you demand that they treat their sick brother or sister with understanding and special consideration. For some children this may be just too much to expect, especially if the strain of treatment continues over a long period of time. Like yourselves, your other children get tired and fed up and need a break. Even if their brother or sister *is* extremely ill, they do not like the fact that they must always take second place. Young children in particular just don't understand.

Illness May Be Their Way of Seeking Attention

Your other children may also become extremely anxious and concerned about their own health. When the whole household concentrates on sickness continually they begin to think that perhaps they are also sick. Sometimes they feel that if they are sick they will get some added attention and privileges. Perhaps they will have more of their mother to themselves—at least briefly.

As your child enters remission and family life is supposed to be more settled brothers and sisters may begin to express their anxiety through a variety of physical symptoms. Some of these, such as headaches, poor appetite, and school problems, are reminders that you may need to make a special effort to give your other children extra attention and to listen carefully to them. This is not a time to panic and believe that they have the same illness as their brother or sister, but it is instead a time to see if additional attention and understanding is a suitable remedy. If you are uncertain your family doctor may be very helpful in determining whether or not all is well. In a few instances brothers and sisters have developed other problems such as asthma and skin rashes, some of which may be caused or aggravated by the stress of their sibling's illness.

Siblings Respond to Security

Most parents want to be honest with their children and help them understand what is happening to their brother or sister. Information must be tailored to the child. Children under age 7 or 8 are not apt to understand detailed explanations about cancer and its treatment. Just like sick children, they can easily misunderstand and become extremely upset if no information or too much information is given. Basically, young children respond to two things. First, they need simple information that they can mull over, absorb, and discuss with their parents. They have to fit the simple details into the framework of their minds and ask questions when they feel the need. They may mix some fantasy with fact even after the most careful explanations have been made. Yet if they are comfortable with their understanding, parents seldom need to worry. Second, young children respond to the security that their parents offer. They are comforted and reassured when they sense that their parents are in control. When Mom and Dad say that it will be all right and that their brother or sister will likely get well again, siblings can feel the reassurance and be content. After age 8 children have an increasing ability to understand more details. However, the fact remains that they too need a chance to discuss their concerns openly with their parents and clear up any misunderstanding. Older children too respond to the comfort and reassurance that their parents offer. Even when the news cannot be reassuring they will appreciate their parents' honesty and the fact that they have not been excluded from knowledge about what is happening.

This continued sharing in whatever happens is important with younger children as well. When you wish to help your other children to understand, there are several ways you can enable them to keep up with what is happening. For example, accompanying their brothers or sisters on clinic visits may help them to work through some of their anxieties so that they can adapt to the present situation. In some clinics, groups and summer camps* are provided for brothers and sisters or time is offered where siblings can play out some of their uncertainties about the hospital, the disease, and its treatment. We have found, for instance, that IV equipment and doctor and nurse dolls are almost as important to the play of brothers and sisters as they are to the play of sick children.

Siblings also gain added security from continuing everyday relationships that were present before diagnosis. Family activities such as trips and outings keep the family together and bring back positive feelings about times past. They provide a rest from the strain of treatment and allow each family member the opportunity to forget current problems for a few moments and be "their old selves again."

In Closing This Section . . .

As we end this section it is important to point out that your awareness of the behavior of your children and yourselves can help you to recognize problems as soon as they begin. Sometimes minor changes in behavior signal the beginning of difficulties. A

* see Appendix E: Siblings' Camps, p. 297.

willingness to discuss problems on the spot can prevent them from becoming more complicated.

In the following two sections we have chosen to pay special attention to the adolescent and to single parents, both of whom have their very distinct problems. In a later chapter we will discuss some of the further difficulties that may arise if a child's disease returns and one or more relapses or recurrences are experienced. If neither the section on adolescents nor the one on single parents has any meaning for you and your child is in remission, you may simply wish to turn to the chapter on long-term survival.

ADOLESCENTS

Adolescents with Cancer
Have Their Own Special Concerns

Adolescence is a time of change—a time of physical, emotional, and social growth. It is a time of frustration, anxiety, and conflict. It is true that adolescents are old enough to understand their disease and its implications, but they do not have the life experience of adults, and this makes it harder for them to live with cancer. Often cancer is seen as a barrier to the type of life that they are trying to lead. Cancer makes them different and can easily isolate them from their friends and acquaintances.

Independence May Be Lost
When Life Changes

Adolescents want to be independent, yet their illness frequently forces them to be more dependent than they were at the age of 11 or 12. Since they lack control over many facets of their lives they must rely on parents, nurses, and other staff at a time when they would desperately like to do otherwise. This dependency creates both frustration and anger. Adolescents are without options. To stop treatment would likely result in death. At the very least there may be withdrawal of approval of the adults upon whom they most depend. As a result adolescents with cancer feel that the disease controls their bodies and their lives. Cancer seriously affects their ability to establish their own identities and values. One 17-year-old girl pointed out that

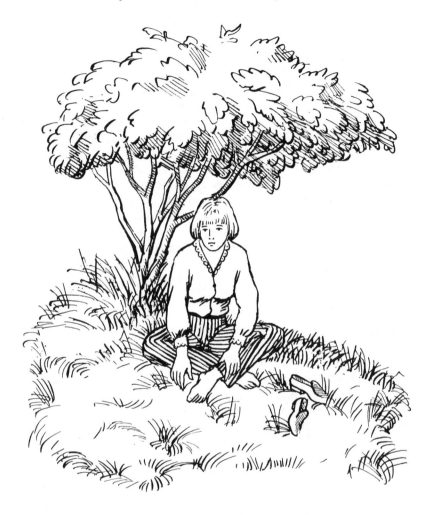

cancer didn't make much sense because she was so young. What did she do in her life to deserve these problems? She had always felt that old people got cancer, and it was so unfair. The hair loss, treatment, and vomiting over a period of 2 years was both upsetting and confusing. She had made plans to attend college and was very active in team sports. She felt that a bright future was ahead, and now, at least temporarily, her plans had to be altered. Cancer meant that she had to readjust her whole life style, and it was most difficult for her to face the controls that were suddenly inflicted on her life and her freedom. It was no wonder that she was angry and discouraged. Her star had fallen, and she just couldn't be the same person that she was before.

Denying

Like most adolescents who are threatened by disease, teens with cancer try to shut out their problems. Shutting out the disease by denying its existence can be very useful. Denial provides time to adjust to the disease and to continue the hope that cure will come. Just as for parents, denial for the adolescent offers a natural respite that relieves the constant strain of a frightening and unwanted disease. When adolescents are encouraged to resume many of their previous activities, their reinvestment sometimes serves to increase their denial. To move in and out of denial is common and allows adolescents to take in information in small bites. Sometimes the message is "Tell me the worst, but don't tell me all of it; do it quickly and then let me turn you off. Tomorrow I may want to hear more, or the same thing again, or nothing at all."

Overcompensating: "Outdoing" Their Peers

Sometimes when you are down there is a great tendency to want to regain all you had before and to do better. Sometimes adolescents try to overcompensate or to outdo their peers. This "outdoing" can occur in a variety of ways. It may be achieved by being at the top of the class or making a dramatic return to sports or gaining special recognition through demonstration of great artistic skill. Adolescents who are successful in overcompensating may reinforce their denial even further. When you realize that denial is normal and understandable your knowledge may help you to support your adolescent. The ability to deny and to drive themselves must be continually recognized as one healthy means that adolescents have to enable them to fight back.

Questioning, Resisting Treatment, and How You Can Help

At some point during the adjustment to prolonged illness and continued treatment most adolescents question themselves just as they question their parents and medical personnel. Like most cancer patients, they ask "Why me?" When they contemplate life further they often ask themselves "Will I die?" "When will I die?" "How do I live with what's happening to me?" Since no answer can be found for these questions adults can only offer honesty, support, and as much understanding as possible. By being there and answering questions in a straightforward manner parents can help the teenagers to temper their need for denial and also help to avoid serious reactions such as extreme defiance. It is not that defiance is so bad, but that in extremes it may be a signal of serious mistrust or uncertainty. Sometimes defiance can get out of hand. We have seen teenagers who have become defiant because they feel a total lack of support from their parents and family. Their reactions have resulted in resistance toward treatment, excessive vomiting, or exaggerated demands for special privileges. Missing appointments, failure to take urgently needed medication, and engaging in activities that have been restricted due to their disease are common examples of defiance. Sometimes when teens are forced to be dependent and very passive these reactions are part of the need to challenge their disease. Being defiant is their way of fighting back. Much of their behavior is related to the anxiety and anger created by their loss of control and independence.

When adolescents are distressed their participation in discussions about their illness with hospital staff and with other teens with the same disease can be helpful. When adolescents feel that they are not alone the support of their peers can be particularly reassuring. Their participation in decisions concerning treatment can also be reassuring. Increasing their responsibilities for even minor aspects of their own care helps them feel that their dependency on others is decreased. Along with more responsibility comes at least some feeling of control and a minor boost in morale.

Physical Changes, Symptoms, Guilt, and Uncertainty About the Future

In addition to adolescents' concerns over their loss of control and increased dependency, they are faced with the following difficulties:

1. *Physical changes.* Adolescents grow quickly, so they may feel awkward and out of proportion. However, adolescence may also bring new capabilities, new skills at sports, and for

some, the beginnings of new beauty. When major changes occur in a teen's body new sexual characteristics emerge. Vanity is a natural part of concentrating on the change and understanding it. Adolescents spend much time both appreciating what has happened to them and worrying about it as well. Acceptance by their peers is all-important, and they worry greatly about how others see and accept them. When their hair has fallen out or they have lost a limb or they have surgical scars that are clearly visible to the world, adolescents with cancer feel different from their peers. They are often so embarrassed and self-conscious that their self-image changes and they lose self-esteem. They feel physically and socially awkward, and the added demands of their treatment program increase their tendency to isolate themselves from peers and sometimes even from close friends. As one adolescent put it, "I have turned into a freak." Missing time at school doesn't help, and fitting back in with the same old social group can be extremely difficult if you don't look and feel the same anymore.

2. *Painful procedures and treatments.* One of the greatest difficulties for adolescents is tolerating painful treatment, especially when it continues over a period of 2 to 3 years or longer. For many, the use of toxic drugs for cancer treatment produces unusual tastes and vomiting, which may continue for 2 or 3 days. Repeated injections and frequent vomiting cause them to become increasingly anxious. After a while this increased anxiety can even make them vomit prior to chemotherapy injections or cause them to have more prolonged vomiting afterwards. Sometimes when drugs are given alternately one causes vomiting and the other doesn't. However, after a period of weeks or months adolescents who vomit from one drug may carry this over to the other drug as well. Adolescents who have these problems may become so upset with clinic visits and treatments that even the smell they encounter on entering the hospital may nauseate them enough to start vomiting.

For some adolescents the use of medications to control nausea and vomiting may not be totally successful. The support of parents and medical staff as well as discussions with other adolescent patients may help in encouraging discouraged adolescents to continue their treatments. The importance of parental support should never be underestimated. For instance, Connie, age 17, a patient with Ewing's sarcoma, reached a point in her treatment program where she threatened to stop weekly injections because she felt she could not tolerate them anymore. Her parents had their own problems and could not offer her the kind of support and encouragement that she needed to reach the end of her treatments. Because of her loneliness and frustration she stopped treatments early feeling that she could no longer carry on. Despite efforts of hospital staff she would not restart and was determined to live with her decision. In a similar situation, but one in which the parents supported their daughter and continued to encourage her right up to the end of her treatments, the results were different. She struggled but continuously sought to gain control of her vomiting and completed her program.

3. *Being a burden to their families.* Practically all adolescents are aware that their illness is of tremendous concern to their parents and to other family members. Many feel guilty about the additional time their parents must spend with them. Others worry about the amount of money their illness is costing the family. Some feel that they must protect their parents from additional worries. For instance, Tom, age 16, was anxious to obtain his driver's licence in order to relieve his family of the need to drive him to the hospital for clinic visits. He was determined to gain as much independence as possible and to make life easier for his parents. Tom's goals were realistic, and he did help. However, other adolescents may try to take on too much or try too hard. It is important that such contributions be sensible and within the capabilities of the adolescents.

4. *Uncertainty about the future.* As part of adolescence, teens look forward to what they may do in future years. For adolescents with cancer, thoughts about the future may be filled with questions about the type of limitations their disease may impose on them. Questions such as "Should I apply for a university scholarship?", "Will I be able to get married and have children?", and "What effect will my cancer have on my own children?" are common. At this point it is difficult to begin to answer these questions because the long-term effects of chemotherapy are not totally understood. It is known that many adolescents with cancer who do survive become active and productive adults. With this in mind it is worth recognizing that they should be encouraged to establish goals for their lives just as other teens do. Without the dreams, hopes, and plans of adolescence, teens with cancer may well become depressed and withdraw. They still

must have the opportunity to live and to do as many things as they are able to do regardless of the anticipated outcome of their cancer.

You Can Never Be Replaced

It is important to remember that because of their desire to live most teenagers with cancer are not preoccupied with death. Most of their energy goes into leading very active lives. Because of their youth most feel that they are survivors and can "beat their disease" even when they experience setbacks. As parents your goal is to help your adolescents to learn and grow in spite of their illness. Their friends are very important, yet they cannot provide the love, comfort, and security that you as parents can offer. A friend may be a poor substitute for a mother or father at times when things are not going well. Friends offer special help and support, but they can never replace you. Your patience, understanding, honesty, and support are needed regardless of what happens.

SOME THOUGHTS FOR SINGLE PARENTS

We hope that you, as a single parent, have benefited from reading the helpful information offered in Chapters 1 and 2 of this book. There are, however, several matters that warrant further attention.

Managing Your Child's Behavior

Earlier we pointed out that some behavior problems only emerge after a child returns from the hospital. Outbursts of anger, bad dreams, irritability, and conflict with brothers and sisters are common. Most single parents find that managing such behavior is challenging, to say the least. Although they know that it is temporary they find that it is hard to be understanding and to continue to set limits at a time when they are worn out from the initial stress of the diagnosis and treatment. As a result, it is worth pointing out that as long as no intense treatment is required most children do reestablish themselves in a month or so, and few have recurrences of behavior problems caused by their illness as long as they remain in remission.

Can You Return to Work?

Any type of continuing treatment means that it will be difficult for you to return to work. This is especially true when your child requires frequent injections or medical procedures. Some parents have found that grandparents and babysitters have been able to cope with bringing a child for clinic visits regardless of the purpose of the visit. Preparation has simply involved coaching the parent-substitute, and unless the treatment program has been extremely taxing both children and substitutes have managed quite well. On occasion, Cancer Society volunteers have also filled this role successfully for children ranging in age from 8 to 17. On most occasions the children have behaved better than they would have if they had been with their parent.

Whether you return to work or not is entirely your decision. The availability of help to take your child to clinic visits is certainly one important factor, but so also is the need for babysitting if your child must be absent from school for long periods. At home, just as in the clinic, your child needs someone whom he or she can talk to and trust. Some children face whatever comes with or without their parents, whereas others need the continuing reassurance that only a parent can offer. Another factor worthy of consideration is family finances and whether part-time employment will provide sufficient income to allow you to manage.

You May Have Delayed Emotional Reactions

On occasion single parents have suffered from stress reactions that occur several weeks after their child is diagnosed. The busy time at diagnosis and hospitalization and the need to care for their children have meant that some parents have not immediately experienced the usual feelings of anxiety, anger, or sadness. Instead they have remained in a state of shock and tried to carry on as if all were well. It was only after they began to feel the total impact of what had happened that they experienced considerable stress. This type of response is hardest for single parents because they still have to cope with trying to return life to as near to normal as possible when they are just beginning to emerge from their own feelings of shock. They are expected to be the manager of the household and be provider, comforter, and stabilizer at a point when they feel that they are "coming apart at the seams." As one mother said, "It was all right as long as Wally was in hospital. I had no time to think. Now I am beginning to realize what it all means. I can't concentrate, and all I can think of is that he may die."

If you feel this way re-read Chapter 1. If you can concentrate sufficiently you may find that some of your questions are answered. It may also be helpful to discuss your feelings with a professional counselor or with other parents who have felt the same way.* If you are able to rely on grandparents, friends, or relatives and can allow them to babysit or help you care for your children in other ways, now is an excellent time to do so. A change, a rest, and a chance to sort out your feelings should make life more bearable. Such a respite may give you the strength to become the family leader again.

You May Feel Tired and Depressed

If you are fatigued do not be surprised if you suffer from short periods of depression. If you are on your own it may be harder to combat your lack of appetite, ambition, and ability to sleep. Fatigue may also make you more irritable, and your ability to enjoy social and sexual relationships may decrease. The same advice as found in the section on delayed emotional reactions applies, except that you may have to make a special effort to become active again, especially when your children rely on you to feed and care for them.

* see Appendix E: Parents' Groups, p. 295.

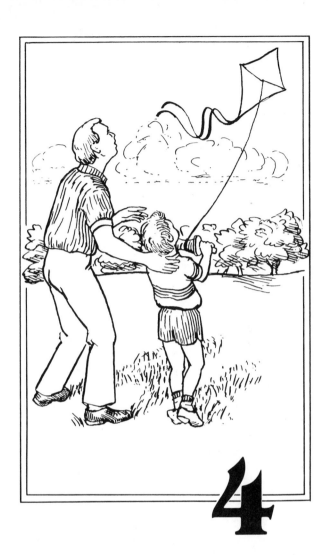

4
LONG-TERM
SURVIVAL

"I am not afraid of tomorrow, for I have seen yesterday, and I live for today."

STOPPING ACTIVE TREATMENT

In the last few years hope has continually increased that children with cancer will live long and healthy lives. If children remain disease-free in a state of remission, active treatment stops. In acute lymphocytic leukemia, for example, active treatment usually ceases after 2 to 2¹/₂ years. The ordeal of taking anticancer medication is over. After medication is stopped check-ups and tests are done several times in the first year and less frequently in the following years. The longer the period that children remain free of disease, the greater the chances of cure. Seven years of disease-free survival is now considered to be a cure.*

For most parents the end of active treatment is upsetting, just as the times of diagnosis and relapse were. Parents feel that a major support is being taken away. They are "losing a crutch." They believe that chemotherapy has kept their children's diseases in remission and that when it is removed relapse may follow. As the time of stopping medication approaches most wonder whether the physicians have treated their children long enough. They also wonder what will be found when diagnostic tests such as bone marrows, biopsies, or scans are done at the time when the treatment is being stopped. If the tests reveal remaining disease it means more treatment and possibly shortened lives.

If you find yourself in this position it is quite likely that you will be anxious too. It is natural to be concerned, and you will likely want answers to a number of questions about the future. Some answers may be found in part of this chapter; others will have to be obtained from your child's physician. If all goes well the rise in your anxiety should be short-lived, and it will gradually decrease through time. Unfortunately, it may never totally vanish because it is difficult to completely blot out the memories and effects of several years of strain.

* George, S.L. et al. "A Reappraisal of the Results of Stopping Therapy in Childhood Leukemia." *New England Journal of Medicine,* 1979, 300, 269–273.

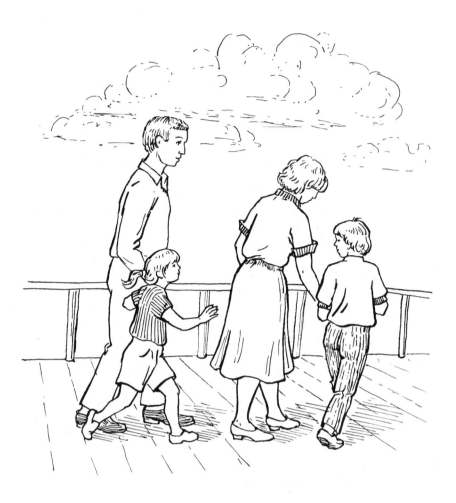

THE YEAR IMMEDIATELY FOLLOWING
THE END OF ACTIVE TREATMENT

After active treatment has stopped many parents gradually relax, but their adjustment will depend upon:

1. Their past experience,
2. Their relationships within the family,
3. The emotional health of family members,
4. The information about survival statistics for their children as given by their child's physician,

5. Their ability to live with the uncertainty that remains.

We have noticed that in the first year or two parents have become very worried if their children are extremely tired, develop fevers or have any other signs or symptoms that might be even remotely connected with the return of cancer. Their watchfulness has also affected their other children, as they have tended to worry that they may also develop cancer.

After 2 or 3 years, most parents tend to be more settled and hopeful. However, some parents have reported that they were still worried about their children even though the children had grown up. Some have suggested that the fear of relapse is never far below the surface.

LATER YEARS

Although our experience is limited at present to a small number of long-term survivors and their families, there have been at least two studies that provide us with additional information. The most useful research available at present is found in a book by Drs. Koocher and O'Malley entitled *The Damocles Syndrome.* * From time to time we will refer to their work in the remainder of this chapter.

In their study of the parents of 103 long-term survivors of various types of childhood cancer, Koocher and O'Malley found that several issues were raised.

1. What are the chances of the disease returning? If cancer returns, what are the chances of children dying?
2. How are children affected? Are they permanently damaged?
3. Will children have difficulties with establishing lasting relationships with members of the opposite sex?
4. Is employment and the obtaining of health and life insurance affected?

What Are the Chances of the Disease Returning?

Before a cure can be discussed, it is important to recognize that survival rates for various types of cancer are based on the

---

*G.P. Koocher and J.E. O'Malley, *The Damocles Syndrome.* (New York: McGraw-Hill, 1981).

results of current treatment. Discussions about cure will vary with the disease. For example, Koocher and O'Malley have noted that 2-year survival is important in non-Hodgkins lymphoma, while for acute lymphocytic leukemia, 2 years after the stoppage of treatment plus 4 years free of disease are required before a cure can be considered. Because information is continually changing it is wise to discuss new developments with your child's physician.

The return of cancer can occur in two forms. First, leukemia may come back or malignant tumors may regrow. Second, there is a risk that new tumors will develop in some types of cancer as a result of using anticancer drugs and specific types and doses of radiation therapy for the treatment of the original cancer. It has been suggested that about 12 percent of all children who survive cancer run the risk of developing new cancer from 5 to 24 years after diagnosis.*

If Cancer Returns What Are the Chances of Children Surviving?

Studies of 5-year survivors from 5 to 24 years after diagnosis suggest that about 80 percent live. This compares with a 97 percent survival rate of the general population for people of the same age during the same time span. Long-term survival and possible cure from relapse depends not only on the type of cancer but also on the length of time after which the cancer has reappeared. For example, in the commonest type of childhood leukemia the chances for survival and possibility of cure are greater if the child relapses after the treatment has stopped. Children who die 5 to 9 years following diagnosis usually die from the initial cancer. In the next 10 years those who die probably do so from a new cancer or from causes unrelated to their primary cancer.

Statistics on their own, given without discussion of children's specific diseases and the course of their illness, are of limited value. This is particularly true of survival rates. Information from 1978 is now outdated. The longer time goes on, the greater the chances for improvement in survival information in almost every type of cancer. There is no doubt that the numbers of long-term survivors will continue to increase, and in fact one group of childhood cancer specialists predicts that by the turn of the century one in every one thousand children in North

* Li, F.P. "Second Malignant Tumors after Cancer in Childhood." *Cancer*, 1977, 40, 1899–1902.

America will likely have survived childhood cancer or will be in the process of treatment for it.

You may profit from requesting current information on survival and recent advances in the treatment of your child's illness. Some cancer centers offer information nights several times per year for parents, allowing them to raise their concerns. If such a service is not available you may have to obtain the information directly from your child's physician. Many parents have been encouraged by the fact that the longer children live the greater the chances that medical advances will be of help, especially if relapse occurs or a second cancer develops later on.

How Are Children Affected? Are They Permanently Damaged?

You have probably been told at some point in your child's treatment that anticancer drugs are very toxic. As well as killing cancer cells, they can affect healthy cells in the body. The liver, heart, and other organs may be affected, depending on the drug and the dose used to treat a particular type of cancer. Each drug has its own side effects, and how they affect your child will depend upon a number of factors.

Radiation can have similar effects. Although radiation therapy equipment has been and continues to be improved, heavy doses or doses to sensitive areas (e.g., lungs) can create both short-term and long-term problems. The age of the child and stage of development is also extremely important. Radiation alone, anticancer drugs alone, or a combination may result in inflammation of organs, failure to develop secondary sexual characteristics, sterility, and long-term deformities.

Many immediate side effects of both chemotherapy and radiation have been discussed in our earlier chapter on treatment. Such side effects are usually visible and temporary. Long-lasting effects such as those just mentioned may not show up for several months or years, yet you probably want to know about them and once again the best source should be your child's physician. However, it is worth noting that in a medical study of survivors reported in Koocher and O'Malley's book there was a low incidence of long-term side effects from chemotherapy. Problems from radiation therapy were greater. For instance, 32 women who received radiation therapy to the abdomen before the onset of menstruation were unable to menstruate and lacked the sexual characteristics of adults. Three women who had their breasts radiated had poor breast development.

The other major group with problems were those who had radiation to the spine. Most of these had abnormalities of growth and development, but as the authors pointed out, as treatment has improved such side effects have become less frequent.

In the same study a small number of patients had physical problems created by surgery, and most managed their deformities and their lives despite their problems.

Most of the difficulties associated with cancer treatment that we have observed have been related to menstrual problems, the loss of a body part, and/or deformity. Several young women have had persistent problems with their menstrual cycles and have worried about their ability to have children. Two adolescent girls have benefited from prostheses to replace muscle loss due to surgery or poor development in their upper leg and buttocks. At least two girls who have had some loss of chest muscle due to surgery have experienced muscular discomfort at times of extreme emotional tension. This has led them to worry that their cancer might have returned, and they have come back to clinic for check-ups earlier than usual. We have had children with amputations, and for the most part they have managed well.

In another example, some 7 years after stopping active treatment one boy still has paralysis of the nerve in his face but has almost totally overcome weakness in one hand left by the removal of a tumor from his upper back. Two girls who have had brain tumors have struggled to overcome learning and memory deficits and a boy has had problems with sports that require a high degree of physical coordination.

There is no doubt that surgery, radiation, and chemotherapy alone or in combination have the potential of causing both long-term and short-term side effects. However, if handicaps do occur your child can be assisted by professional staff to learn to live with them or in some instances to overcome them.

Long-Term Adjustment. When Koocher and O'Malley studied how 117 long-term survivors adapted to life in general they found that better than half were managing well. Another one-quarter had mild problems, and about 22 percent experienced moderate or severe difficulties. Of these just under 3 percent were severely affected.

Those who had the most difficulty reported shock and distress at the time of diagnosis instead of relief at the fact that the disease could be treated. As their distress continued they also worried about the disease returning and tended to withdraw from their usual social contacts.

Those who were distressed tended to feel dissatisfied with themselves, were more anxious, had more times when they were sad and depressed, and had more problems in relating to other people than those who did well.

In total, the survivors had a wide range of reactions. Some felt privileged to survive, some wanted to help others, and some felt that they were special to have been spared. Most looked to the future, realized that they could die, but did not feel closer to death. Interestingly, about 20 percent felt that their families were of little help and noted that people in the family usually did not want to listen to their problems or understand their feelings about their illness.

Although these findings represent children from years past, they bring to mind points that are worth remembering.

1. Children do work hard to make up for their handicaps or deficits.

2. Opportunities exist today to help children more with both physical and emotional difficulties than at any point in the past. Some children may require professional help. For instance, several adolescents have consulted with clinic staff about their worries regarding social and emotional problems associated with side effects related to treatment. These have included anxiety about being left behind by friends because of loss of time at school and uncertainty about careers due to their needs for special considerations. Relationships with the opposite sex have also been a concern because of deformity or possible inability to have children. Sometimes simply having access to information or someone to share their concerns has helped greatly. If your child requires such assistance, allowing him or her to seek it will likely make life easier for you as well.

3. Parents now are better informed about their children's problems and how to help them than parents of the past. If you can listen to your child and provide the emotional support required you may help reduce the emotional problems that might occur later on.

Will Children Have Difficulties with Lasting Relationships with the Opposite Sex?

We have seen a number of young people who are worried about their relationships with the opposite sex, and particularly their ability to perform in marriage. Problems have ranged from lack of development of breasts or other parts of the body to loss of teeth from radiation to the jaw. So far our observations of small numbers of long-term survivors suggest that adolescents and young adults have tried to compensate for their difficulties and have not let developmental problems ruin relationships with the opposite sex. Several have requested and received special help to obtain prosthetic devices or sought medical and social advice about their fertility and participation in sexual activities.

In one study of 124 long-term survivors from the mid 1970s the major problem seemed to center around marriage. Only about half of the subjects had married, and about one-quarter of those over the age of 20 suggested that cancer or disability had hindered their marrying. Koocher and O'Malley's findings were similar. Almost half of those in their group who were between the ages of 21 and 37 had not married. Koocher and O'Malley concluded that the more physical problems women had, the less apt they were to be married. Single men, on the other hand, tended to have more psychological difficulties.

For those who did marry, the major concerns of their spouses were associated with the health of their offspring and with sexual functioning. In most instances these had been explored and resolved prior to the time of marriage. Only two of sixteen marriages were childless, and those with children reported no serious child health problems.

Are Employment and Obtaining Life and Health Insurance Affected?

We have seen a few instances of discrimination against cancer patients who are seeking employment or who are applying for life insurance. Once again the Koocher and O'Malley study offers the most specific information available to date. In 60 long-term survivors over the age of 18 they found that about 40 percent experienced some form of discrimination related to employment or military service. Almost half had been denied life insurance at least once, and eight had been forced to pay higher premiums. About 64 percent had some form of life insurance at the time of the study. Most of the sample had some form of group health insurance, but only a few had individual health policies, and most excluded illnesses related to a history of cancer.

WHAT ARE THE EFFECTS
ON SIBLINGS?

In all four areas of concern discussed so far findings suggest that the overall adjustment of survivors is positive, and for most parents this should be reassuring. However, one remaining question does arise: What are the effects on siblings? Brothers and sisters are very much affected.

Our observations are that siblings feel jealous at times and left out at others. They run the risk of being scapegoated by upset parents, and some siblings become so distressed that they do poorly in school. One study notes that siblings of children with cancer are more prone to injury and to being isolated from friends. They are more anxious than their peers and worry about confronting the family with negative feelings. Koocher and O'Malley found that in 51 brothers and sisters of cancer patients born before cancer was diagnosed in their siblings (a) they remembered the treatment time most clearly; (b) at least one-quarter of them had been jealous; (c) about one-third worried that they too might have cancer; (d) some had been upset at not being allowed to visit the hospital, had difficulties in school, or had been forced to defend their sick brother or sister; (e) a few had felt contaminated by cancer and rejected by friends; and (f) some had to be a support to their parents.

When we consider this information the material found in earlier chapters of this book becomes increasingly important. Parents must pay attention to the feelings of other children and provide emotional support to help them face the outside world and to dispel their anxieties about developing cancer.

BONE MARROW TRANSPLANTATION:
ONE ADDED HOPE FOR THE FUTURE

Before closing this chapter it is worth mentioning that some children with cancer, particularly those with leukemia, may be able to benefit from bone marrow transplantation. This procedure allows bone marrow cells to be donated by a person—usually a sibling or parent—whose blood matches specific criteria. Marrow is taken from the bones of the donor and is introduced into the body of the cancer patient. Usually the patient's body is prepared for this procedure by giving specific drugs and radiation to the entire body. The patient's own marrow becomes inactive, and eventually the donor's marrow creates new cells that are totally disease-free.

Children who undergo bone marrow transplantation are usually placed in isolation to protect them from infections for a minimum of 3 to 5 weeks. If all goes well they are then transferred to outpatient care. During the first year after transplantation they may be required to wear a mask and observe certain precautions to prevent infections.

This procedure is a major step for both parents and children. The hospitalization and the uncertainty of the outcome are agonizing. In the adult type (myelogenous) leukemia, for example, 60 percent of transplant patients can expect to have a long-term disease-free survival and it is hoped that the majority will be cured. In the commonest type of childhood cancer (lymphocytic) 45 to 60 percent of children with this disease who receive the bone marrow transplantation will survive for at least 3 years free of leukemia.[*]

Transplants may be unsuccessful because the donor's cells are rejected. The complications from graft-versus-host disease and from infections may be so serious that they are life-threatening. Nevertheless, at present bone marrow transplantation is the best option for a child with leukemia who is no longer responding to drugs. Unfortunately, at present where there is not a perfect tissue match with a brother or sister bone marrow transplantation is extremely difficult.

As time goes on, more will be learned about ways to transplant from donors who are less closely matched than siblings or other family members. New methods will also be employed. In fact, in some centers, the patient's own bone marrow is being frozen during remission and given back to the patient later on. So also will new methods be developed to control or eliminate graft-versus-host disease. As medical knowledge increases bone marrow transplantation will likely become a major contributor to long-term survival, particularly in leukemia.

---

[*] Gale, R.P. & Champlin, R.E. "Bone Marrow Transplantation in Acute Leukemia." *Clinics in Hematology*, 1986, 15, 851–872.

IN CLOSING

As persons who have worked with and cared for patients and families, our greatest ambition would be to expand this chapter considerably in a few years' time. Long-range survival of children with disorders such as leukemia, Hodgkin's disease, and Wilm's tumor continue to improve with each passing year. As one parent pointed out, "We at least have our son well and we are enjoying life. Even if cancer returns at some point later on, maybe then new drugs will have been found so that he will be ensured of a permanent cure."

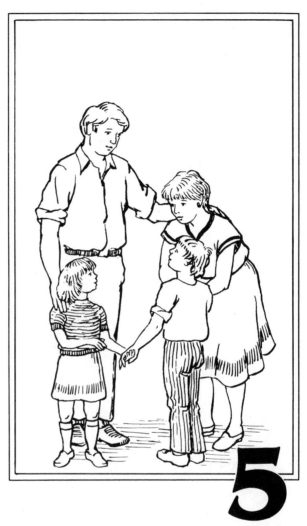

5

RELAPSE

THE MEANING OF RELAPSE

The first relapse comes as an enormous blow to everyone in the family. It means that the dreaded signs and symptoms of cancer have returned. In the case of leukemia malignant cells reappear in the bone marrow and in the blood. With tumors the malignant mass may begin to increase in size or there may be metastasis or spread of tumor cells to another part or parts of the child's body where a new tumor begins to grow.

WHAT USUALLY HAPPENS WHEN RELAPSE OCCURS

Relapse often means that your child will require hospitalization in order to start treatment. In leukemia maintenance therapy will be stopped and induction treatment started again. Induction treatment may mean that a new combination of medications given in higher doses will begin. You may be familiar with most of these drugs, as your child received them at the time of diagnosis. However, the order, method, and frequency of administering them may be quite different. A few new medications may also be added, and the intensity of the whole treatment program may be much greater than at any point in the past. No doubt your child's physician will explain the whole process in detail. Most parents are so upset by relapse that they need to hear the explanation more than once.

The goal of this aggressive approach to treatment is to eliminate the malignant cells as quickly as possible and thereby have your child's disease reenter a state of remission. In many cases of leukemia a second remission can be achieved and maintained with continued treatment that lasts up to 3 years. Once again the goal is to keep your child in a permanent remission. If a further relapse follows later on it is usually more difficult to induce another long-lasting remission without resorting to other procedures such as bone marrow transplantation (see Chapter 4 on long-term survival).

If a tumor begins to grow again or new ones appear your child's physician will likely consider various approaches. Surgery may be indicated to remove the growth or growths. This may be followed by radiotherapy and possibly chemotherapy. As with leukemia the medications used may be the same as those previously given to your child, but they may be given together with different drugs and in much higher doses. In some cases only radiotherapy or chemotherapy may be indicated to control the tumor growth or to eliminate it completely. The treatment may be brief or may extend over a period of 2 or 3 years depending on the location of the tumor and the type of cancer involved. Your child's physician will explain the treatment program and should offer you some indication of the success or failure of past experiences in treating cases similar to that of your child.

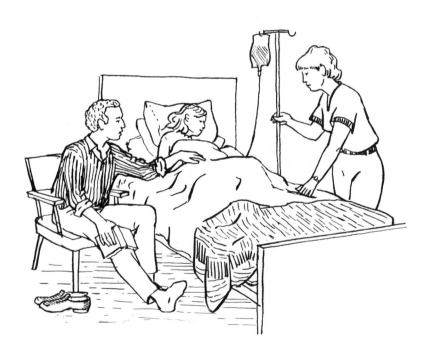

THE IMPACT OF RELAPSE

"Relapse was a struggle for us . . . a time for new worries . . . a need to renew hope."

"For us relapse was not a shock because of our faith in the doctors . . . . Our standard question was 'What do we do next?' or 'Where do we go from here?' "

"Relapse was the beginning of the end . . . oh God! . . . . Our worst fears came true!"

These three responses represent the variety of thoughts and feelings that parents have when a child's illness relapses. Many parents worry that the road will be downhill from relapse on, and in some cases their concerns are realistic. Somehow they must find the strength and courage to allow themselves and their children to go on living. They must find a sufficient measure of hope to buoy them up at a time when it is easiest to feel defeated and totally overwhelmed. The following sections examine some of the changes in their lives that others have experienced and offer some advice about how to cope.

HOW RELAPSE STRIKES

Remission was a period of time when your child appeared well and was able to gradually resume many or all of his or her usual activities. Quite likely your family gradually settled down, and the daily routine became more normal and acceptable. You probably understood the nature of your child's disease but perhaps did not fully recognize and accept its implications. In fact, many parents report that the period of remission increased their hopes as well as their denial. They found themselves holding back any anxieties in favor of believing that this remission could last forever. They became certain that their sick children would grow up and live normal lives. These reactions and beliefs are very understandable and very common.

There is no doubt that relapse is even more difficult to bear when it follows a very long remission. The first relapse often comes very unexpectedly. It may strike suddenly with little or no warning at a time when your child appears well and has no obvious signs or symptoms of disease. Often the first sign of trouble arises when a mother senses that her child appears ill or is reverting back to some behavior that reminds her of a time just prior to diagnosis. Theresa, age 8, was a very active swimmer, yet one day she just sat by the edge of the pool and cried. Her behavior quickly reminded her mother of a very similar situation that occurred just before the diagnosis of Theresa's leukemia. On routine examination the next day at the clinic abnormal cells were found in Theresa's blood. Just as in Theresa's case the first real sign of relapse in leukemia is usually detected when routine blood work is taken during a child's regular clinic visit. In most cases it is necessary to perform a bone marrow aspiration to determine whether this is truly a relapse or a common reaction to infection.

In the case of tumors children may have no symptoms or may experience discomfort, pain, limping, weakness, shortness of breath, or any number of difficulties. Sometimes the only sign of trouble arises when the physician feels an unusual lump or mass during a routine physical examination. Following such a discovery it may be necessary to proceed with further examinations including x-rays and bone scans.

FEELINGS AT RELAPSE:
HOPE, GUILT, ANXIETY, AND ANGER

Hope

With the sudden knowledge that your child is in relapse or has had a recurrence of cancer you may be overcome with severe disappointment and despair. We have pointed out that relapse does not necessarily mean that your child's death is close at hand. Others may have told you the same thing, yet you believe that all hope has vanished. If you feel this way, then you cannot go on from this point without changing your thoughts and feelings. To subject your child to further treatment without believing that it may be helpful would be senseless. But consider this. Who can say that there is not enough reason to continue to hope? It is true that we cannot believe in something that is known to be impossible. However, how can you be certain that it is impossible for your child to survive this disease? Researchers know that cancer can be a killer; however, they defy this fact by continuing their research in hopes of finding cures for every type of cancer.

A personal experience with an 11-year-old boy and his family has firmly established for one of the authors the belief that there is always room for hope even when death seems inevitable. Otto, age 11, was lying in the intensive care unit supported by a respirator. It was strongly felt that the respirator should be withdrawn because Otto was fighting it, his brain tumor was out of control, and he should be allowed to die peacefully. After considerable discussion with the family and medical personnel it was decided to gradually discontinue all life support systems. Otto was relieved because he hated being hooked up to the machine. Once he was off the respirator Otto's condition gradually improved, and 3 weeks later he was able to go home as a patient in the Home Care Program. This was a situation in which everyone including Otto believed that there was no hope for his survival, yet Otto continued to live.

When you do lose hope, in most instances you need to rekindle it for your own sake as well as for the sake of your child. This may be a tremendous challenge for you and for your family! In many situations aggressive treatment can lead to remission and possibly to cure, but the path may be painful. You and your child may require considerable encouragement to make it through. It is certainly reasonable for you to feel sad and disappointed, but relapse is rarely a time to give up. In fact, parents who have been through the experience tell us that they could not allow themselves to abandon all hope even in the face of the poorest prognosis. Instead, when they considered their children's need for intense treatment they realized that some of their expectations for the future were unrealistic and needed to be altered, at least temporarily. For instance, one child had relapsed during his second year of remission. When he had 2 months of chemotherapy left before he completed his 3 years of post-relapse treatment, his mother commented, "We might get him off drugs, but I am not counting any chickens before they are hatched." She was hopeful, yet she knew that much time and successful treatment were required before she could be sure that her son would survive.

Guilt

Just as at diagnosis and during any time of intense treatment, parents have felt guilty because their children's disease returned. They have felt that somehow they had failed and let their children relapse. Once again many have been haunted by the feeling that an earlier discovery of their children's diseases would have made a difference in their recoveries. Relapse also has reawakened a yearning for answers. Questions related to the importance of other possible causes such as urea insulation in their homes, industrial pollution, contaminated drinking water, or inheritance of the disease from other relatives have returned to plague them.

You will probably have some of the same concerns. It is important for you to keep in mind that this disease is very unpredictable, its cause is seldom known, it often returns suddenly, and in some cases very little, if anything, can be done to prevent either its occurrence or reoccurrence. For example, one mother felt guilty because her son had gone through extensive surgery and his cancer metastasized very soon after. She felt that she could have prevented his pain and suffering, but no one could predict that the cancer would spread in spite of the surgery. Most parents have a need to do what they feel is best for their children. Nothing can make them feel more inadequate and helpless than a disease like cancer. When you are faced with a child in relapse somehow you have to resolve your guilt and maintain control. You must recognize that you do not have supreme power over life and that no one has the right to hold you accountable for an illness like cancer, not even yourself.

What's Ahead: Anxiety Affects the Whole Family

New experiences create new worries about what is ahead. Relapse brings parents to what one mother described as the edge of the cliff. She was desperately worried that her daughter would tumble to her death and the family would be shattered by her loss. Although most parents are less dramatic and the shock of relapse is said to be less than the one that strikes at diagnosis, the worries about the future are real. Many of the concerns described in Chapter 1 are alive again, and the anxious behavior shown at diagnosis has a habit of repeating itself. Without dwelling at length on the impact of new stress on parents, it is our intention instead to show by example how their distress and the return of the illness combines to affect children.

Ingrid, age 8, suffered a relapse of her leukemia and began an intensive chemotherapy program. Although her parents supported her emotionally, she was upset by the injections and nausea and vomiting that followed. Her mother was uncertain about putting Ingrid through such suffering, so when she was given chemotherapy injections in her mother's presence she became extremely upset. Ingrid's anxiety continued, and at home the family's uncertainty about her well-being led her parents into allowing Ingrid to sleep in their room. Ingrid became very dependent and clinging even at home. Exploration of her behavior revealed that she was worried that if her parents moved her out of their room she might die in the middle of the night and no one would be with her.

Malcolm, age 11, was upset by the return of his cancer. He saw that his mother was upset and seemed reassured when she received help from hospital staff. He tried hard to control what was happening to him and continually asked questions. His uncertainty combined with his parents' anxiety had a "halo" effect on his brothers and sisters, and they became distressed as well. His anxiety increased when he suffered from symptoms of his illness and changes in his body. The more he suffered the more he wondered whether he should hope for a time free of treatment. He became very distressed when another child in the clinic died, and he was reminded of her death each time he passed her home on the way to the clinic.

When he relapsed Marty, age 12, became extremely aggressive. He expressed a desire to get even with the staff for hurting him and ran away and hid when brought to the clinic for treatments. He began vomiting before needles were given, and it continued for many hours afterwards. He told the staff, "I'm scared, I hate having needles, I don't care if I die." His mother had great difficulty comforting and disciplining him. She was frightened by the treatment and by everything that was happening.

Barry, age 7, relapsed and was hospitalized. His mother tried to reassure him. She told him that all would be well, but she continually hovered outside of his room. The more she hovered the more anxious Barry became. The least change in routine upset him greatly. He became irritable at the slightest discomfort and demanded more and more medication for pain. Both Barry and his mother were so upset that they were unable to help each other cope with the uncertainty ahead.

In these four cases there are several common observations worth noting.

1. The children were intelligent and perceptive. They sensed their parents' uncertainty. They knew that their parents were having a tough time managing the situation.

2. The change in their illness was perceived as a major threat to maintaining their daily lives. All probably worried that they would die, and some expressed their worries directly.

3. The children showed their anxiety in many ways. Ingrid clung to her parents. Malcolm tried to control his treatment and worried about the future. Marty vomited more than most children and ran away from treatment. Barry was very apprehensive if anything changed, and his pain increased at the same rate as his uncertainty.

4. Relapse brought new treatment programs that were distressing. These increased the children's anxiety and created new demands for parents to provide additional support and comfort. Anxiety was compounded. Treatment added a new burden on top of the burden of not knowing whether the future held life or death.

How Can You Control Your Anxiety? Most parents struggle with varying degrees of success to gain control over what is happening. Some become increasingly fatalistic. A supreme being, usually God, has a plan mapped out and survival rests on fate. Some find comfort from their faith. They believe that their children will live or continually pray that their children "will be spared." Some have struggled to be more optimistic and have become strong believers in the power of positive thinking. Clearly, there has been no universal solution. However, most parents have recognized the need to resolve at least some of their uncertainty and regain as much self-control as possible in order to provide strength, comfort, and guidance to their children. What a difficult task this is when parents are mourning the loss of the remission that held the greatest hope for a long and normal life for their children.

We believe that:

1. Most parents benefit from discussing their feelings. The examination of personal strengths and deficits as part of the process helps many find new hope and courage.

2. Many parents take heart from their past ability to manage. "If we can cope with the diagnosis then we can cope with the relapse." It is true that overcoming the initial shock and the strain of treatment prior to remission strengthens many parents. They learn to cope. Many parents do this very well.

3. Partners can be a tremendous asset if they can be in tune with each other's feelings and be honest enough to share their thoughts and feelings with each other. A parent team is needed to manage what is ahead—a team that works together and provides unity and direction in the face of a nasty and sometimes devastating illness.

4. Even when parents are uncertain they can still offer love and security. It is reasonable to be concerned about the future. It is reasonable to let children know that you don't have all the answers. However, it is essential that you let them know that you and your partner are going to be there every step of the way. It is also important that you let them know that you expect them to receive the necessary treatment, that they can express their feelings about it, and that you hope the outcome will be positive. In other words, you can "call the shots," but you must also "deliver the goods." When parents are strong children are usually strong too.

As we mentioned earlier, anxiety is mixed in with other feelings. Children who are discouraged often feel sad. Rather than repeat a review of children's responses as found in Chapter 1, we recommend that you re-read that section. We will focus in the next section on anger and how parents can help children express it.

Anger

It's All Right to Feel Angry. For most parents anger accompanies guilt and sadness. They and their children have struggled through difficult and painful times only to feel defeated by relapse and have their lives turned upside-down again. They have every right to feel angry. Just as at diagnosis, most anger is directed at God or hospital staff or relatives. Anger may be stimulated by unusual jealousy aroused by the sight of healthy children or reminders of times when life was free of this problem. Some parents have told us how they inadvertently directed their anger toward their family and even toward their sick children if they misbehaved. Their anger just upset their children further and made a difficult situation even more unbearable. No wonder parents are angry at this time. They are often worried and tired to the point of being "worn out." They just don't have the patience or the energy to cope with any added pressure.

Children Have Angry Feelings Too. Many children may also feel very angry and disappointed. Relapse may make them think that all of their previous tolerance of treatment has been useless. Those who suffer most have often been told that they would stay well if they took their medications and endured the painful treatments. As a result their trust in their doctors and their parents may be shaken. Relapse meant that their lives became restricted once again. Just as during earlier periods of continued treatment, their play activities, school, and friendships were all seriously affected.

At relapse you may find that routine visits to the outpatient clinic become increasingly difficult. The number of visits will likely increase and may bring back unhappy memories as well as a return to painful procedures, tests, injections, and medications. For children whose treatment program has been light or nonexistent because they have been disease-free since the time of diagnosis, relapse introduces a totally new and frightening experience. Parents have told us that they and their children have both questioned whether this more intense treatment is actually worthwhile if the cancer has come back anyway. Many wonder how their children will manage without losing the will to keep struggling and fighting back against the disease. Just as for any child who is treated aggressively, injections will make some of them sick and the procedures can be painful. Some also run the risk of experiencing numerous physical changes including the loss of hair or the gain or loss of weight. A few may undergo surgery that results in disfigurement. General weakness, irritability, nausea, and vomiting may also be associated with new bouts of radiotherapy and chemotherapy. When children do not feel well or are self-conscious about changes to their bodies some miss considerable time at school, lose contact with their friends, and reduce involvement in sports.

Some parents have found that illness and frustration have caused their children to be very demanding and at times quite unreasonable. For example, David, age 6, became increasingly upset at receiving injections. He lashed out at his mother and punched and swore at her. When he was left alone in the room and allowed to slam doors and act out his anger he was able to calm down. Children do need opportunities to react to their frustration and anger. As you may recall from Chapters 1 and 3, hospitalization and any type of continuing treatment can increase your child's anger. Kyle, age 8, relapsed and was hospitalized. He was frightened by the hospital and the treatments and missed his friends. He was most upset at missing soccer games. On numerous occasions he became very rude and made unreasonable demands on his mother and the hospital staff, particularly when he was reminded that he must remain in the hospital. With the help of the child life worker Kyle was able to work through this anger in play therapy, and he gradually settled down. Sarah, age 14, was also admitted to the hospital following her relapse. The separation from her friends at school and the results of treatment including hair loss were very distressing. Gradually she became withdrawn, bitter, and hostile. During injections and medical procedures she would fight to the point of exhaustion. She would settle down only when medical and nursing staff were firm and reassuring. Even then her anger lingered, and when the nursing staff attempted to do even minor nursing procedures she would try to bite them. She behaved like a much younger child, and her fear and anger mixed together were so strong that it was hard for the staff to help her overcome it.

Sometimes anger may be expressed indirectly, and this is especially true at relapse. Joan, age 10, hid her anxiety, sadness, and anger by giggling during examinations and difficult treatments. She never showed her anger at the clinic, but tended to be irritable at home. When she was told that she would lose her hair because of the intense chemotherapy she increased her aggression toward her older sister, who was her usual target. After she worked out her feelings she calmed down and accepted the need to wear a wig and receive continuing treatment. Gradually, with the help of clinic staff, she learned to express her feelings directly.

In another case Bart, age 9, was upset by conflict at home and by the renewed need to treat his leukemia due to relapse. At home he communicated little with his parents, but he was very aggressive and dominant at school. He was involved in several fights, and when he and his sister were alone he would continually punch her. Bart's anger had to be released, and he chose what he believed to be the safest route. He knew that hurting his sister and the children at school would probably go unnoticed. He knew that anger toward his parents would mean punishment, and he worried that anger toward the doctors might make them less willing to treat him.

How Parents Can Help Their Children Overcome Anxiety and Manage Anger

In earlier chapters, and particularly in Chapter 3, we noted how parents can help children to overcome their anxiety and release their anger. You may wish to re-read this information. Remember that your child

1. Has every right to be upset.

2. Needs to know what is happening and should be allowed to make simple choices about food, visitors, rest times, etc.

3. Needs you and the consistent emotional support and guidance you can offer.

4. Will benefit from praise to reinforce success when he has released anger constructively and controlled his anxiety.

5. May find physical outlets helpful—punching bags, throwing games, hammering, and playdough. Perhaps the most innovative game was invented by 10-year-old Jay, who was confined to bed. He made himself a giant target from newsprint and had his parents tack it up on the wall at the foot of his bed. A few newspapers were placed on the floor and Jay used much effort to shoot spit balls through a plastic tube at the target. This game may not be desirable for everyone, but it helped Jay.

6. May be helped by music, books, and sharing thoughts and feelings with other children.

7. May be frightened and upset. Remember that anger tends to increase when children feel that they have lost control. Punishment should probably be a last resort. Reassurance, security, and minor rewards are more apt to restore control both for you and for your child.

PAIN: ONE SOURCE OF DISTRESS FOR CHILDREN

Anger is one form of distress arising from frustration with parents' behavior and with the side effects of illness and treatment. Controlling distress from parents' behavior is dealt with in other sections of this chapter, so let us turn to the control of distress related to treatment. One major source of distress is pain. Pain arising from cancer itself often creates intense discomfort in or over muscles, joints, and bones. Such pain can be controlled by the skilled use of medication and can be at least partially checked by increasing a child's level of relaxation.

When pain arises from injections or procedures such as lumbar punctures or bone marrow aspirations the problem is a bit different. Relaxation can be increased by the use of simple exercises, and a child's overall level of anxiety can be reduced by play therapy, which allows the child to become familiar with the procedure and the equipment required. Local anesthetics given at the point of aspiration or puncture can also help. When painful IV injections must be given frequently the problem increases. Familiarity with the equipment and procedure through doll play can be of some help, but the strain of the procedure can be great. If you recall, we have dealt with this at some length in the chapter on Remission and Treatment. The case of Paula serves as a reminder of the intensity of the problem. After many injections she began to scream hysterically and then cried and cried. She could not tolerate any more. The following section may offer one solution to the problems of children like Paula so that their level of distress never reaches these extremes.

One Real Possibility for Reducing Pain— The Hickman Catheter

It is easy to recognize that aggressive treatment programs make a major impact on everyone, especially if many injections are required. For this reason some cancer treatment centers have begun to use a device known as a Hickman (tunneled right atrial) catheter. Although insertion of the Hickman requires a surgical procedure and a general anesthetic, it provides for much less pain and suffering than when repeated IV injections are given. Usually the catheter is inserted under the skin of the chest and attached to a main vein. When injections of medications or other substances are required they can be made directly into this catheter rather than into the child's arm. Thus the problem of the painful search for small veins and possible spillage of medication from them is avoided.

Hickman catheters can be left in place for many months providing they are properly maintained. Usually a solution of heparin or saline is used to keep the catheter clear of blood and special disposable caps are replaced regularly. If the catheter is properly looked after these children can continue almost all of their normal activities without serious risks of infection.

For children facing major treatment programs the Hickman has reduced their suffering tremendously so that they are much less upset by other procedures and much less distressed by chemotherapy treatments than are children who receive regular intravenous injections.

THE ADJUSTMENT OF SIBLINGS

Brothers and sisters will also feel the impact of this relapse. Anxiety, sadness, anger, guilt, and jealousy are common sibling reactions. Suddenly everything must once again revolve around their sick brother or sister, and this can be frustrating. The family routine is again disturbed, and often their plans must be changed to accommodate their sick brother or sister. If this occurs frequently you can begin to understand why they feel jealous. They may also see their sick sibling missing school, staying in the hospital, receiving presents, and having lots of attention from Mom and Dad and other relatives.

Most brothers and sisters feel sad and some feel guilty because they believe that they did or said something that may have caused their sibling to get sick again. Sometimes these feelings may be difficult for parents to detect. For example, Jack, age 7, was angry that his brother Peter received some money from relatives for finishing eighth grade. Jack, being younger, did not receive any similar gifts. In anger he wished that Peter would get sick again. Three weeks later Peter was readmitted to the hospital and Jack felt responsible.

Brothers and sisters may also be very anxious about developing cancer themselves. They have seen so much that they may conclude that since their sibling's cancer came back then perhaps they might also get cancer. Some worry that their parents might also develop cancer. They need to be reassured that they cannot catch cancer and that it cannot be passed on to them or to their parents.

When your children are faced with these worries you must take the time to talk with them and explain what has happened to their brother or sister. If your explanation is simple and conveys your desire to still love and care for them, they may be helped to deal with their own feelings and reactions to the sudden changes in their family. Your words can also help them to realize that you are sad, upset, and concerned about their brother or sister. It is reassuring for them to know that you feel sorry that you cannot be at home when you are needed at the hospital. This knowledge will help them to find added courage and patience to face the rough times ahead. Allowing relatives whom they like to fill in and stay with them may be helpful. Your willingness to take turns with your spouse so that you can be home with them from time to time may also make life more bearable.

Understanding, honesty, reassurance, love, and support are needed as much by your other children as they are needed by your sick child. Parents tell us that it is terribly difficult to be sensitive to all of the family's needs and still have enough energy and patience remaining to deal with all of the problems that may arise.

ADJUSTMENT TO LIVING

If you are like most parents you may feel overwhelmed by the suddenness of the changes that are necessary to allow you to care for your sick child again. If your child has been in remission for a long period of time these changes may be even more difficult. Family life has been turned upside down, and it takes a tremendous effort to maintain any normal family activities. Some parents wonder whether or not their families will ever be the same again. Some have stated that relapse felt like a turning point in their child's illness from which everything seemed to go downhill. Other families have faced relapse as a challenge and they have drawn closer together in a concerted and determined effort to fight the disease in every way possible.

Most parents find that relapse increases their emotional stress and their level of fatigue. Some have suggested that relapse was like starting all over again with more drugs, more side effects, and more procedures. They felt that many of their initial anxieties from the time of diagnosis returned. Their stress level rose sharply, and some believed that their child's relapse created more stress than the actual diagnosis, because they were shocked to learn just how uncertain and unpredictable cancer could be.

You will probably find that relapse brings back all the painful feelings that you associated with the threat of losing your child when he or she was first diagnosed. You probably wonder how you will manage and whether or not you will survive yourself. You may be one of those people who have been uneasy anyway, and relapse simply confirms your doubts. Some parents live in a state of chronic tension that never really subsides. On the other hand you may have buried the thoughts of relapse at the back of your mind, removed from possible recall. If so relapse will hit you harder. You may need time to sort yourself out, and you may need help to recover your grip on your thoughts and feelings. We have often found that one or two counseling sessions can be an asset to parents who have totally rejected the thought of relapse. We have also found that parents with this response tend to have stronger emotions and may have to grapple with feelings of deep and renewed bitterness. These feelings need to be discussed and released in ways that will not be harmful to you, your spouse, your sick child, and other family members.

Stresses That Affect Many Families

In preceding chapters that dealt with diagnosis and remission we discussed the variety of stressful factors that parents faced. Many of these stresses may have diminished or subsided over time, only to be reawakened and become very real again during the time of relapse. Some stresses may become even more significant than at any other time during your child's illness. It is important to remember that each family experiences different kinds and amounts of stress. One situation may be extremely stressful for one particular family while for another family it may not be a problem at all.

It may be helpful to examine some of the common stresses confronting your family at this time. Knowing about them and recognizing their impact may be of value to you.

Changes in the Roles of Family Members. Once again parents are challenged with new or different roles. Mother may have to resume the job of being home, taking the child to the hospital, or remaining there to be the major source of comfort. Father may be forced to become part-time homemaker and overall manager of life at home. Relatives may be called into service to help, and everyone feels the strain of renewed illness.

Financial Difficulties. Since diagnosis some families have been under constant financial pressure that has remained or continued to accumulate. Relapse may add to the problems as new financial pressures arise from costs associated with increased treatment. *

Need for Better Understanding of the Disease. Changes in your child's illness may require you to develop a greater understanding of cancer and its impact on your child. New learning may be needed to understand new terms, the names of new drugs and their side effects, and new schedules for treatment. Your child's physicians and nurses can be helpful, and you may have to ask them to write down this information so that it can be taken home for further study.

* see Appendix E: Financial Concerns p. 295–296.

Questions About Treatment. Many parents wonder whether new research findings or new drugs are available to help their children. They worry that the cancer treatment center may be out of date or falling behind centers that are touted as being more progressive. A renewed questioning and search for miracle treatments are common. If you feel this way your child's physician should be prepared to discuss the matter with you. Such discussions may result in feelings of security or may lead you to request consultation with another center. You must feel secure about the treatment program and believe that you have selected the best center and the best physician.

Challenge to Faith and Hope. As discussed earlier in the chapter, relapse tends to challenge the faith and hope of many parents. Some parents find that discussion with someone outside of the family such as a social worker or clergyman may help. At the very least such discussions can help clarify your questions and help you arrive at your own conclusions about how you are going to live with your child's disease from this point forward.

Problems in Relating to Others. The strain of knowing that your child's life may be "on the line" again makes it difficult to know how much to tell others. Involving friends and family often means receiving renewed help and emotional support. For some parents, though, it may mean a renewal of problems seen at diagnosis when friends and family were upset and frightened and tended to pull away, resulting in abandonment at a time when support was needed most.

Positive Aspects of Stress

Although most of this chapter focuses on major stresses and their negative impact, it is worth mentioning that not all stress is negative. Some parents have learned a great deal about themselves, their children, and their spouses and have undergone considerable personal growth. Many have changed their values and set their priorities on finding happiness in living their daily lives together. As one parent explained, "Today we have each other, for how long we do not know, but then again no one really knows." Relapse creates a need to reassess, reexamine, and renew families. It is a time to come together and regroup to fight back in the face of the threat and uncertainty that lie ahead.

THE ADOLESCENT PATIENT

The Importance of Symptoms

When relapse occurs adolescents are most apt to be concerned about their new symptoms. These may appear as weakness, pallor, new lumps, fever, or pain. These symptoms are uncomfortable and frightening, and they bring with them threats of more treatment to come. Some of this treatment may be similar to past experience while some may be new and anxiety-provoking.

Symptoms frequently remain the focus of an adolescent's adjustment for the rest of the disease. If symptoms are mild most normal activities can be continued, but some adolescents may be more upset than their symptoms seem to warrant. Much depends on how the adolescent interprets what is happening. As some experts have pointed out, the quality of life of any two adolescents with cancer will vary so much with the impact of the symptoms that even though they may have the same amount of time left to live one adolescent may be irritable and ill while the other may be back at school and participating in sports. This can occur because the symptoms of cancer are actually less severe or because the more active patient interprets them as being so. If the severity of symptoms increases, the same sort of variations will occur as other factors such as level of anxiety, tolerance for pain, and amount of parental support provided become increasingly important.

The Beginning of the End or New Ordeal?

Parents may see relapse as the beginning of the end or, as one parent put it, "a sinking feeling begins." For most adolescents the immediate concern is less with the end result than in beginning treatment again. More visits to the hospital, more diagnostic tests, and several bouts with injections must be faced before most adolescents dwell at length on survival. For some, relapse means a lengthy hospitalization complete with new attempts to deny what is happening and loss of place and self-esteem. Sadness, depression, and struggles for independence may be prominent if treatment is taxing or adolescents are extremely ill. In some cases upset adolescents will act out, and a very small number of distressed adolescents may become self-destructive. For most anxiety will increase, and some will become more religious or place much importance on super-natural beliefs. When parents are confronted by such behavior they must consider what adolescents need from them. Parents want to help, but sometimes it is hard to know what to do. In the remainder of this section we will examine the problems of adolescents in more detail and provide some useful sugges-tions for parents.

Losses

At the time of relapse many of the observations and concerns noted in the previous chapters on diagnosis and treatment hold true. Adolescents are prone to the same feelings of loss of con-trol, of self-esteem, and of social place. They are also confronted with the problems of disfigurement, mutilation, and other per-manent or temporary side effects that may accompany either disease or treatment.

Feelings and Ways Adolescents Respond

Anger. Feelings of anger are most common at this time because changes in the adolescents' lives are disrupting, upset-ting, and annoying. Parents are often excellent targets because it is easier to be angry with them than with the doctors and nurses, who are seen as the sources of pain and suffering but are difficult to approach. After all, they do control the treat-ment, represent authority, and have the potential for "getting even." Remarks such as "Sure, they want to help me, but all they ever do is hurt" are common. Most parents recognize that it is quite reasonable to protest. If they were in the same situa-tion they would strongly object to having their lives temporarily or permanently ruined. The only problem is that some parents are hurt or confused by their adolescent's anger and lose their ability to be effective. Sometimes when this happens adoles-cents' desires to rebel or escape override both reason and the usual controls that parents maintain to help their teens. As a result angry adolescents may stop taking oral medication or refuse or physically resist medical procedures.

Denial. Sometimes adolescents try to deny the reality of the meaning of relapse. In order to do this some tend to focus their concern on a specific symptom or procedure. For example, if a leg is swollen devoting much time and interest to it may help them to temporarily avoid examining the other possible meanings of relapse. Similarly, complaining about bone marrow tests and protesting against the treatment program may help take the focus away from the cancer and provide avenues through which adolescents can gain some control.

Denial, like anger, comes and goes. After treatment begins again or the intensity is increased the real meaning of more treatments creeps back in. For some, new drugs mean a continued hope for cure, while others believe that their chances for survival are severely reduced. Much depends on the messages given by hospital staff and family and the extent of physical illness. Adolescents who feel sick tend to be less hopeful and more concerned about whether or not they will ever be well again.

Facing Reality. Despite their desire to deny, most adolescents are very much aware of the realities of their illness. Most physicians make every effort to tell them directly, even if they have to impart small amounts of information during several meetings. At times adolescents may not want to hear what they have to say or can only accept small amounts of such threatening information. Sooner or later many will allow the reality to seep into their thinking, at least for short periods. Most will admit to being frightened and choose specific people with whom to share their concerns. For instance, one or two staff members may be selected because they are seen to be less threatening than parents or other adults.

Sadness and Depression. The reality of cancer, worries about the future, and losses of social place that come with relapse all combine to make adolescents sad. If they have many symptoms and are hospitalized the dragging on of the treatment process may make such sadness more permanent. Often adolescents display symptoms of depression. These include the inability to laugh or smile, loss of appetite, constipation, and difficulty sleeping. Restlessness, boredom, and irritability are all common, as is the necessity to temporarily withdraw from social contact. These symptoms tend to vanish fairly quickly for most adolescents when they experience improvement in their physical health, learn there is genuine hope for their survival, and are allowed to return home.

Independence Versus Dependence. A continuing struggle to be independent often accompanies the recognition that life may be shortened. For some adolescents hospitalization and illness can breed dependence, which is prolonged, protective, and reassuring. If adolescents remain in the care of hospital staff and begin to rely heavily on them, they become inactive and listless to the point where it is difficult for them to return home. To do so can become a "leaving of the womb" and a frightening removal from the safety of the hospital. Even though the hospital has been a source of pain and discomfort, the routine has become acceptable. Isolation from family and friends is more desirable than risking a return home. Home means new demands, less personal care, and exposure to the frightening routine of outpatient treatment.

Being Different. Going home means a return to social circles where former positions have been lost—perhaps for the second time. As one teenager who returned to school put it, "I feel like a cancer freak. Everybody looks at me because I'm different." Another adolescent with a marked disability couldn't bear going to church because everybody watched her and felt sorry for her. Another tried returning to school and found that most of her former friends ignored her. Since she had missed the last part of her year due to relapse and her friends had moved on, their behavior made her feel "like a second class citizen, a real 'dummy.'" When teenagers feel this way it is important that they discuss their feelings and frustrations with a counselor or someone else who can be understanding.

Acting-Out and Self-Destruction. Some experts have pointed out that for a tiny number of teens problems in adjusting to extensive surgery and the return home may lead them to destroy surgical repairs or to threaten their lives. Fortunately, these responses are infrequent. They are usually caused by deep-seated anxiety about losing control and fearing death. Teens who behave this way need psychiatric help immediately.

Increased Anxiety About Death. The intensity of treatment, anxiety of parents, and new knowledge all tend to increase adolescents' anxieties about death. Sometimes fears are realized through dreams. For example, Armand, age 16, dreamed that he was in a box in the morgue. He was not dead, but he could not tell anyone. He cried out because he wanted to go to the hospital clinic where people knew he was alive.

At other times anxieties may creep into everyday life when adolescents resist treatment and try to escape, much like the adolescent patient we describe later in the chapter on dying.

Although discussion of one's own death is very frightening, some teens are able to do so directly and find it helpful. Others tend to find indirect discussion less threatening and will ask about other patients or talk about concerns that others have about death. By being indirect, reality and anxiety are kept one step removed and are therefore more easily tolerated.

Religious Beliefs and the Supernatural. When teens think about death they frequently reexamine their feelings about religion. As 17-year-old Betty suggested, "I believe there is something up there . . . everybody prays . . . when my parents push it (religion), it is hard to accept . . . praying helps at first. I stopped them from making me go to church . . . now I go once in a while just to keep on the good side."

Like many adults, teenagers often incorporate superstitions and myths into their thinking and behavior. Good-luck pieces, religious medals and good and bad omens are faithfully considered but seldom talked about, especially with parents.

It is important for parents to recognize that adolescents do think about the control that external beings or superstitions have over them. Some find such beliefs helpful and supportive, while others may be confused or upset. Adolescents may need help to sort out the mixture of fantasy, reality, and feelings that shape their thinking. Sometimes these beliefs have a marked influence on adolescent behavior, and some influences may be very positive. For example, some adolescents want to help other people and will go to great lengths to do so. On careful examination it may be revealed that the underlying reason is part of their need to bargain with God so that they will get better. Bargaining can help them to feel less guilty or to feel that they have genuinely helped another person. Sometimes a problem arises when adolescents experience increasing disease and become intensely angry that God has let them down or cheated them.

What Do Adolescents Need at This Time?

Adolescent years are very difficult for most parents, and treating adolescent patients can be a genuine challenge for hospital staff. There are several areas where adolescents require support, understanding, and sometimes help from others outside of the family. Some of these areas are discussed in the following paragraphs.

Clarification of the Facts and Fantasies About Cancer.
Just as most adults speculate about what causes cancer, so
also do adolescents. Such speculations may include the effects
of chemicals in food, exposure to pesticides, and viruses.
Speculations may also border on myth and fantasy and related
thoughts and feelings. For example, 15-year-old Carmen
thought that God had singled her out to be ill because she was
the strongest person in the family. Norma, age 16, believed that
God was surely punishing her for the "wild" life she had led. The
best approach to dealing with the possibilities is to have
hospital staff discuss the realities of what is known about the
causes of cancer. As a parent you should make every effort to
ensure that this happens.

The Role of Family and Friends: Sorting Out Feelings.
The most difficult place for many adolescents to express their
feelings is in the presence of their parents. In the teen years,
just as in early childhood, adolescents of each sex experience
periods when it is difficult to relate individually to either Mom
or Dad. These difficulties change at various points, and for a
while one parent may be in greater favor than another. Negative
feelings toward either parent may last for several months and may
be most intense when parents are strong-willed. For example,
Carolyn, age 16, was extremely angry with her father, who was a
stern disciplinarian. She felt she could never win against him.
Members of her family seldom discussed feelings other than
anger, and up to the time of relapse she was unable to tell
anyone how she felt and what she needed. She was at an age
when it was easiest to be close to her mother, so that under
stress her mother became the major support. Some months
later her negative feelings about her father reduced, and he
played a more active role in her care.

Since many families avoid discussing strong feelings,
especially sadness, it is difficult for adolescents to include
parents at times when they must admit their frailties. At relapse
many are in turmoil and are plagued with anger and sadness.
They don't feel good about themselves, and although they need
reassurance and understanding it is hard to obtain it from the
authority figures in their family. If family members do not ordinarily share their feelings should parents try to change? Can
they genuinely do so in a short period of time? Quite likely such
changes would be extremely taxing and difficult to accomplish
quickly. Many families need continuing help to begin to talk
about subjects that have been embarrassing or threatening.

They require preparation in order to behave differently so that they can support each other. Right now may not be the time to change. Adolescents often find that any change is threatening, especially when they feel that they are losing control of everything else. It is also hard to close the natural distance between parents and teenagers, and it is not usually desirable to try to do so rapidly. Parents may find that they already have ways to support their adolescents that are helpful, and if further support is needed it can be provided by others who are outside of the immediate family.

For families who have open systems of communication the task for parents is easier. Quite naturally the distance between parents and adolescents is smaller, and as in Carolyn's situation there is usually one parent who is seen to be understanding. This parent can be trusted and can be a person with whom a son or daughter can share at least some feelings. If a teen becomes sicker, the tendency to trust such a parent or parents will probably increase. This happens because the teenager becomes more dependent on others for physical care and because dependence forces him or her to regress and behave like a younger child.

In families where feelings are not shared and relationships with parents are very strained, increasing dependence may or may not change relationships positively. If adolescents remain sad and withdrawn, or act out, there are several possible avenues through which help can be obtained. Often a hospital social worker or counselor can help. This person can assist adolescents to express their feelings and to come to grips with hospitalization, treatment, and if necessary, progressive disease. Parents may also receive help because counselors can provide suggestions aimed at improving parents' knowledge about supporting their adolescents during relapse. Sometimes parents and siblings benefit from continued counseling aimed at helping them to understand and express their own feelings.

In some hospitals special adolescent groups for teens with cancer have been developed to provide emotional support. These groups help adolescents to realize that they are not alone and provide a nonthreatening place where thoughts and feelings can be shared away from parents who might find them to be bizarre, alarming, or hurtful. In our hospital such a group has helped adolescents who are receiving injections to reduce the nausea and vomiting that accompanies such treatment. Even preliminary vomiting has tended to decrease when adolescents are able to express their anger and sadness with peers.

Sometimes close friends may offer adolescents emotional support that is quite different from the support provided by parents yet similar to that offered by an adolescent group. Parents often recognize that friends help to provide relief from the monotony of life with adults. Most realize that friends may improve adolescents' outlooks on life. Even though parents may not be convinced that the influence is always positive, they recognize that friends offer a special viewpoint, communicate on the same wavelength, and are allies in maintaining an adolescent's will to fight off the disease.

In addition to talking and being comforted adolescents need to have other ways of expressing their feelings. For instance, 15-year-old Michael was able to talk about his leukemia more easily when he drew pictures of the hospital, 17-year-old Marilyn wrote poetry about her feelings, and 14-year-old Anna kept a diary. Nancy, age 16, remained involved in sports. She played basketball as long as she was able to run, even in the face of increasing illness.

The Adolescent's Self-Image

Just as adolescents have feelings about how others affect them, they also have feelings about themselves. As we mentioned in Chapter 1, they worry about the future and how others see them. The process continues and intensifies at the time of relapse. Being different is distressing, and being the reason for disruptions in the family adds guilt to the anger and sadness already present. Many adolescents believe that they are responsible for being sick and for forcing families to change vacations, go into debt, and remove their siblings from the home to be left with relatives for days or weeks on end. For persons who already feel that they have lost much through changes in appearance and mobility, these added feelings of responsibility are enough to send them into at least a minor depression. This is especially true if parents continually make it known that the family is suffering and that daily sacrifices are being made because of their illness. As one teenager said, "I wish I weren't in the hospital. It makes my mother tired, transportation is difficult, the rest of the family can't see me, and I worry about what all this is doing to them."

If your adolescent relapses much of your behavior will be governed by day-to-day changes in his or her physical and mental state. Changes in symptoms and reactions to tests and treatments will influence whether you are sad, angry, or lighthearted. The behavior of your son or daughter will also change frequently. Despite these shifts in day-to-day feelings, there is a strong likelihood that an underlying philosophy or common family attitude toward illness and treatment will persist no matter what happens. For instance, some adolescents may be tough and cynical and want to beat the disease. Their tough exterior is a means of protecting themselves and a way of fighting what is happening to them. Others may joke and laugh in the face of disaster and allow very few people to really know how they feel. Some may become philosophical and use highly intellectualized discussions as a means of escaping and forgetting their problems, at least temporarily. Such discussions also offer protection because the real issues are avoided. Others may be very dependent and seek additional comfort and help. Such dependence may mean that they receive a lot of affection and caring. When this happens they may also feel that they don't really have to face the reality of their illness because others are taking care of them no matter what happens. Still others may continually deny and behave as though nothing is the matter. On occasion strong denial that persists may result in a shock to adolescents who must face unpleasant realities later on. Each philosophy or attitude and accompanying behavior is closely tied up with how the family is coping. It is usually the intensity of such behavior rather than the philosophy that changes as the family struggles with cancer. The basic philosophy only changes when major information is received that will affect the outcome of the illness.

No one can dictate how any person should respond to cancer. As parents, however, you have a responsibility to try to manage your own feelings and support and encourage your son or daughter. Relapse is probably the most difficult time of all. At a time when you are worried that this may be the beginning of the end you are required to care, to share, and to try to understand the thoughts and feelings of a person in turmoil. It is a time when you still must have rules and continue to provide the structure necessary to support your son or daughter regardless of what happens. If you have a relationship with your adolescent that is reasonably successful you probably shouldn't try to change it. For goodness sake, don't pull away because you are uncertain or upset. If, however, relationships are strained and you and your family—including your adolescent with cancer—need help, ask your family physician or other hospital staff for it. Help received now may make whatever happens in the future easier for everyone.

SOME THOUGHTS FOR SINGLE PARENTS

Most Single Parents Feel Powerless

The devastation described earlier in this chapter is especially difficult for single parents. The threat that a child's life may be shortened is hard for couples to face and almost unbearable for many single parents. We have found that single parents tend to believe that they will face the worst possible outcome and that they may "fall apart" themselves. They recognize that their family system is fragile and quickly raise many questions about medical treatment and changes in work and living patterns. For some, recurrence of disease brings back memories of early disruptions in family life and the stress that everyone faced at diagnosis. For others, the situation may be worse because the initial hospitalization was short and the treatment then was relatively simple. The reality is that most single parents worry. They worry about how they will face what happens if their child deteriorates, how they will manage to keep working and bring a child for more intensive and frequent treatments, how they will be able to explain what is happening to their child, and how they will be capable enough to continue to manage the daily lives of their family.

Because many single parents feel inadequate, especially if separation and divorce has been recent, the personal challenges are more intense. Most feel the burden deeply, most are anxious, and some become depressed. If you are in this situation you have every right to feel upset. You probably feel angry that you are left on your own to cope with the problem, when at least 50 percent of it should belong to your former partner. Questions such as "Why me?" or "Why us?" may mean even more to you than to other parents because you bear a double burden. You can expect to feel even more powerless at relapse than at any point since diagnosis. Quite likely you will believe that almost every aspect of your life is being controlled by others.

How One Parent Faced Her Problems

When you feel that you have lost control and are overwhelmed it is very difficult to regain your composure. When Cynthia, the mother of Debbie, age 8, was in this position she found that it was helpful to list her problems and to try and solve each one independently. By reducing her problems from one gigantic, overwhelming dilemma to several individual ones she found that each was less threatening. By concentrating on one at a time she could come up with satisfactory solutions. The following paragraphs describe some of her problems.

Should She Continue to Work? Initially, Cynthia thought that she would have to stop working and that she had no other options. After thinking about it she decided that she did not really know enough about what was to follow to answer the question. She only knew that her child's leukemia had returned and that an injection program would follow. Since she had some paid leave coming she decided that she would use it in the following week so that she could bring her daughter to the hospital for further tests and the beginning of more intensive treatment. By the end of the second week she had decided that she would try to change her hours of work to allow her to start at noon rather than at 8:00 a.m. This meant that she could come with Debbie on a regular basis and still continue to work. Her employer agreed to allow her to try this for 3 months because she was such a valued employee and because much of her work was done independently.

Although this was not a permanent solution for Cynthia it meant that she had at least found a temporary means of continuing her income. Such a solution gave her time to make a more permanent decision about her work that was based on actual experience rather than on speculation.

How Could She Cope with the Worry That She Might "Fall Apart?" This problem was extremely trying for Cynthia because she felt that she was a weak person. She partially blamed herself for the break-up of her marriage and believed that she was unattractive. She also felt that she could never care for a dying child because she was so sad and frightened. Cynthia was on her own, since her parents were elderly and her in-laws lived in another city. She had, however, faced the diagnosis reasonably well, had continued to work steadily, and had taken time off work only when her child required check-ups. Because she was so upset clinic staff counseled her. The social worker and nurse-practitioner helped her recognize that she had several strengths. First, she had not "fallen apart" so far. Second, she had maintained family life even though she had suffered personally. Debbie had adjusted well to her illness as had her other daughter, Karen, age 10, and her son, Greg, age 6. She was a good mother who cared a great deal about her children and managed the family well. Third, she had not had time in recent months to test out her attractiveness to the opposite sex and so did not know what men really thought about her. The staff certainly didn't look upon her as an ugly or unattractive person. Fourth, and most important, Debbie's medical situation was not without hope. Although her prognosis on chemotherapy was only fair there was a chance that she could survive. The completion of donor compatibility testing for bone marrow transplantation offered one other possibility for cure. During these discussions Cynthia responded by recognizing her strengths and realizing that even if the possibilities for her child's survival were exhausted she had time remaining to prepare herself for her loss. This was reassuring to her, and she showed renewed confidence in her ability to help Debbie face the treatment program.

How Could She Manage Her Children When She Hurt So Much and Felt So Tired? At one point just after Debbie's illness relapsed Cynthia thought that she just didn't have the strength left to manage the family. Even the simplest household tasks were difficult. Because of the strain of the moment Cynthia had lumped everything together in her mind. She was dreaming of piles of dishes and cleaning the house each night in her sleep. She worried about not finding the time to pay bills, cut the grass, weed the garden, or do anything else around the house. Once Cynthia wrote down what she must do she began to organize the tasks in order of importance. She soon recognized that a simple schedule of daily activities approached in this manner could help her begin to plan her life.

Along with the organizational problems Cynthia had to grapple with some very real questions about how to care for her children. She worried about what to tell them, whether or not she should treat Debbie differently, and how much responsibility she should give to Karen. After careful consideration she decided to tell Debbie that her leukemia was back, that it was a miserable disease, and that she hoped that the treatments would make it go away. She told her the treatments would hurt and would make her ill but that Cynthia would try to comfort her and help her as much as possible. Debbie accepted her mother's explanation and was at least temporarily satisfied.

As Cynthia learned more about the treatment program she decided that it was quite likely that there would be times when she would have to treat Debbie differently. For instance, following injections Debbie was likely to have episodes of vomiting and might miss a day or two of school. Despite this Cynthia was determined to keep Debbie in school as much as possible and to discipline her when she needed to be punished. Cynthia seldom spanked Debbie anyway and decided that her current practices of depriving her of television or treats and isolating her when necessary should continue to be effective. She also decided to explain to the other children what was happening to their sister and told them exactly how determined she was to keep order in the house.

After much careful thought Cynthia decided that all of her children could do more to help out at home and enlisted Karen's assistance in doing slightly more housework than the younger children. All three children responded to their mother's suggestions, and it was agreed that if Debbie was sick for a short period she would be allowed to catch up on her work in a day or two and that the rest of the family would help her. If she was ill for a long period they would discuss what to do at that time. Although Cynthia was able to find some solutions for her problems they were not all lasting or perfect, and some plans required revision later on. In fact, problem solving was a difficult process and one that helped Cynthia learn more about herself and her capabilities. She also found that even though some problems were solved life did not always become easier, because new ones emerged. For instance, she soon learned that when Debbie was ill after injections she vomited for several hours, so Cynthia had difficulty getting to work at noon. Luckily, she found as a babysitter an older woman who could tolerate such problems, and this helped greatly. Later, this woman became invaluable when Debbie missed school due to a severe infection. She provided an added dimension of security that Cynthia desperately needed in order to continue to manage the family.

In closing this chapter, then, the message from Cynthia was that tackling her problems one by one made her into a more effective and efficient single parent. She became a mother who learned to guide her family through the difficult and complicated period of her daughter's relapse. What she learned may be of value to you.

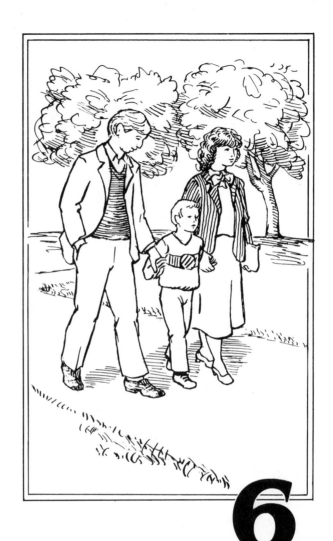

6

CHILDREN'S
KNOWLEDGE OF
DEATH

THE PURPOSE OF THIS CHAPTER

When cancer threatens a child's life the other children in the family are exposed to the possibility of the loss of a brother or sister. Many parents have wondered what children think and feel about death. You may have similar questions; if so, this chapter will be helpful to you. Your knowledge will then help you to assist your children as they learn about death as part of their normal growth and development.

Customs and rituals have evolved through history. Therefore, we will begin by providing some background information and then proceed to describe the meaning of death for children at various ages.

HOW THOUGHTS AND FEELINGS ABOUT DEATH HAVE EVOLVED

Hiding Death

Death is an upsetting and bad experience. It is something to be avoided at all costs. We and our parents before us have been part of the North American pattern of hiding death. For instance, in the past 25 years North American cemeteries have changed from clusters of stone cairns and tombstones to plain green fields or "havens of eternal rest" complete with names like Rose Lawn, Forest Lawn, Rest Acres, and other titles implying a garden-like setting free of all evidence of death. Death has become something that happens to others, an event of old age, or the outcome of a tragic accident.

How Longer Survival and Death Rituals Have Changed Our Expectations

As children of the recent past many of us have grown up without being exposed to death. It is no wonder that we are uncomfortable. We are part of society's move away from the country to the city and from large to small families. Death has moved too, and death in the hospital has become much more common than death at home. Death rituals have shifted almost exclusively to the funeral home, and wakes held in the family's parlor have all but vanished.

These changes have been accompanied by changes in our expectations. We expect everyone, especially children, to live long lives. Advances in medical care have revolutionized our outlook. For example, in 1900 just over half of all the deaths in the United States were those of children under age 15. By 1974 only 7 percent of all deaths were in this age group. Overall childhood deaths had dropped a remarkable 46 percent, and the numbers of young adults and middle-aged persons who died decreased as well. Because so few children die we want to ignore the fact that there is a possibility that a child cannot be cured of an illness. Apart from knowing that children may die from accidents, cancer, leukemia, and infant mortality, we are very easily lulled into believing that death belongs to the aged.

The Rebirth of Death as a Subject for Discussion

In the 1970s North American society experienced a rebirth of two forbidden subjects—sex and death. The works of Dr. Elisabeth Kubler-Ross and others helped the public and professionals (especially health workers) to find a new interest in death.* In the early 1970s courses in death and dying became very common. Suddenly professionals realized that dying persons should be able to talk about death and that few professionals were trained to listen. Ministers for years had learned to deal with death by "seat of the pants" experiences and by trial and error. Doctors, nurses, social workers, psychologists, and other professionals were in the same boat. Gradually the public also began to recognize that dying persons were often rejected and that it was

*See E. Kubler-Ross, *Questions and Answers on Death and Dying.* (New York: MacMillan, 1974).

all right to speak about death. The beginnings were not easy. In one prominent church, for example, a series of sermons on death upset the congregation so much that by the third Sunday only one-third of the people attended the service. The congregation found that it was too threatening to accept the fact that cancer, heart disease, and other disorders could cause death in youth and middle age.

Fortunately, this reawakening and realization has led authorities toward providing care for the terminally ill in home-like settings called hospices. Programs have also arisen in hospitals to improve the quality of life of the dying and to provide palliative or comforting care when cures are impossible.

HELPING CHILDREN UNDERSTAND DEATH

As parents we must help our children to recognize that death is a part of life. We must help them face death not just as seen in the make-believe world of television and books, but as an experience that will happen to them, their parents, friends, relatives, and pets. We must assume this task as people who want to share in both the joys and sorrows of life. However, most of us are poorly prepared for this task and have much to learn.

It is worth recognizing that death can be frightening for both children and adults. It is true that children encounter and accept the death of leaves, trees, and objects around them and do not seem to be greatly moved by death on television. However, the death of a grandparent or even a pet is much more personal and upsetting. Such a loss is a new experience, and most children need their parents' help to understand it. The more gently and realistically parents can approach the subject the better. Rabbi Grollman, a pioneer in research toward understanding children and death has suggested that if parents avoid the subject children's anxiety mounts and their imagination has the chance to run wild.* We can be most helpful when we appreciate how children at various ages think and feel about death. This includes beliefs about death itself, death as something that happens to others, and death as it applies to themselves.

*E. A. Grollman, (Ed.). *Explaining Death to Children*. (Boston: Beacon Press, 1967), pp. 6–7.

UP TO AGE 5

Within the first few years of life and particularly from the fifteenth month on, children develop a sense of self-worth and try to learn how to rely on themselves. They depend heavily upon their parents and mimic their thoughts and feelings. As a result, toddlers worry most about being separated from them and especially from their mothers. For toddlers, dying simply means separation, and the final loss of a mother or close relative can produce anger, worry, and withdrawal. It is not usually until age 3 or 4, however, that children begin to discuss death and to think about it in their own simple way.

At about age 4 children begin to play act death, and death in their games is completely reversible. You can be dead one minute and alive the next. Dead people are capable of eating, seeing, thinking, and moving around. Death may be associated with darkness, violence, evil, and sleeping. The world of death is confusing and changing, and things like sewers and ditches and "boogey men" can become part of children's thinking. Consequently nightmares are common, and many young children are afraid of the dark.

Despite its threatening quality death must be faced, and it should be included in children's stories and play. One authority stresses the value of fairy tales because they bring tragedy into the make-believe world of the child. Fairy tales may include deaths and injuries, but they are free of the seriousness of adult life. In fact such tragedies are so much a part of everyday life in the story that children can accept them without directly relating death to themselves. Play is similar, and make-believe worlds offer relief from the intensity of love, hate, and learning, which are so much a part of everyday life. In play, just as in fairy tales, death can be confronted and is free of hurt and sorrow. When they have been faced in play the same qualities of death can be carried into real life. When the dead are believed to be living, then dead relatives and pets can continue to be a part of children's lives. This allows them to think and talk about a subject that can be very threatening.

Because children can quickly move in and out of both fantasy and reality, thoughts of death cannot always be harmless. Death has a darker side, and children recognize that it can make people feel sad and frightened. They too are frightened, and their natural tendency to associate darkness and evil can creep into their thinking and upset them. Worries about death can also lead them to link their beliefs into relationships with parents and sometimes in a very primitive way with God. Young children may see death as punishment or a way of getting even for their acts of wrongdoing.

Because children in this age range can easily be confused or distort what has happened to a dead relative (frequently a grandparent), it is important that we as parents help them to be realistic without completely interrupting their need for fantasy. We must be prepared to talk about what children feel and know and be reassuring to them as well. The examples that follow illustrate the importance of such reassurances.

Some Case Examples of Young Children Whose Relatives Have Died

When Jimmy, age 4, experienced the death of his 7-year-old sister his parents discussed the loss with him, and all seemed to be going well. About 4 weeks after her death, he broke out in a rash and screamed hysterically. After much comforting Jimmy told his parents that he was upset because he expected his sister to come back to stay in her room and play with him. Another child, Bobby, age 3½, refused to go to sleep after the death of his grandfather. In the middle of the night he had bad dreams that made him wake up screaming. After some discussion he told his father that if he went to sleep he thought that he would be like Grampa and die.

When she was 4½ Susan's father died. When her mother drove her out to the cemetery Susan talked about her father on the way, but on arrival became upset. She was worried that there were no stores to supply her father with food and clothes and there was no one to help her father get out of his box. She was afraid that he might trip if there was no one to look after him. Another child, age 2½ wanted to know who shot her father because people had to be shot to die, just as she had seen on television.

Children Can Learn About Death from a Variety of Living Things

It is in this formative period that children develop patterns of behavior that will be used at times of crisis later on in life. They also begin to develop religious beliefs which continue to be

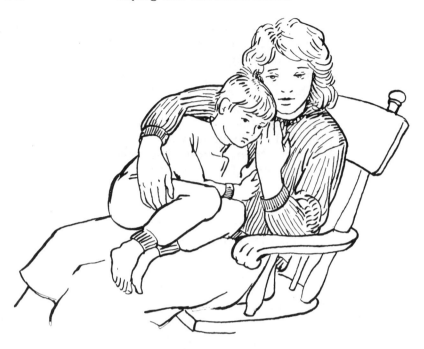

formed throughout childhood. Sometimes during this period if no family deaths are encountered it is worthwhile for parents or grandparents to teach children about death by discussing the loss of a favorite pet or the finding of a dead bird.

In one family the parents told us how the death of a dog gave everyone the chance to discuss their sorrow. The children planned a small burial service, and family members talked about the happy times and affection that the pet had brought to each of them. The parents had the opportunity to tell their children that death was permanent and that everyone would die some day. In other situations parents have used leaves, flowers, and the death of other living things to explain the cycle of life. One family had a flowerbed full of dead guppies. Their graves were marked by crosses made of plastic straws placed there by their young son. His feelings of loss led to an easy and natural exploration of the meaning of death.

As parents we should remember that it is quite all right for children to see our sadness and sorrow. Children may have a much shorter attention span and may be put off by continued mourning by their parents, but they mourn too. They need to be allowed to be sad or angry and shouldn't be judged if their sadness is short. In many cases their initial response to a family loss may be fleeting and matter of fact. They need time to mourn and to come back and ask questions. They need parents who will listen, share in their sadness, and speak openly about what has happened.

Some Guidelines for Parents

If you have young children the following guidelines may be helpful.

1. Let your child tell you about death.
2. Listen to your child's questions. When you answer, keep your reply simple and to the point.
3. When you have answered your child's questions, stop.
4. Your child is naturally curious, so relate death to things he or she understands.
5. Do not associate sleep with death.
6. Do not say someone was taken away or that God took him.
7. Do not say a dead person has gone on a long trip.
8. Do not just say someone was sick. Carefully explain in very reassuring terms that many people become sick but only those who are very, very ill may die.
9. Do not talk about the "loss" of someone. Children may worry that if they "get lost" they too will die.

When someone dies we must help our children feel that they are still needed and are important. Despite our own sorrow we must help them go on playing and living as part of the family. If you are secure even when you are grieving your children will be secure also. Remember that it is all right to cry. Like happiness, sadness is a part of life that children must experience. When children are distressed by death for reasons that you do not understand you may find to your surprise that you can help them by participating in their play activities. Sometimes a nursery or grade school teacher can help. However, if your child is terribly distressed counseling may be needed even though it may be upsetting for you to have to ask for such help.

AGES 5 TO 9

Children begin to develop a greater understanding of death as they grow older. Their feelings of sadness are stronger, and they often show much sympathy for the dead person. Death gradually switches from being within a body that continues to live to being a final separation from a person who is loved and missed.

Ages 6 and 7

At age 6 or 7 magic is still very much present in children's thinking. Children may associate death with ghosts, witches, and monsters and may be worried about them hiding in the closet or being present in the dark. If you recall, we talked about how young children fear separation. They worry about being taken away from their mother more than anything else. At age 6 or so children begin to worry more about being mutilated or destroyed. Mutilation anxiety takes over as the biggest fear. As a result death becomes frightening and dangerous because there is a worry that some type of dark, scary being will come and take them away.

As part of this anxiety, and attempts to master it, boys, especially, want to know more about death and bodies. The knowledge of detail seems to help them to have control. Fantasy life is also used to confront death. Death is often play-acted in war and in violence, and the gory details may be discussed with playmates.

Along with concern about loss and sadness may come worries about the death of a parent or themselves. Some children worry about growing old and struggle to relate time to aging and death. This is very difficult, because children still have much trouble understanding the meaning of time and may picture their parents to be very old at the age of 35.

Age 8 and 9

As children approach age 8 or 9 many become more secretive and keep their thoughts and feelings to themselves. They begin to realize that those who die have less chance of living again. They may begin to worry more about their own death, and their anxiety about it may be channeled into fantasies with heroes and adventure. Such anxiety may also surface quickly at the time of the death of a family member or friend. Many children begin to try to reason out the meaning of life, heaven, and life after death.

Since death continues to be associated with fears of retaliation or getting even for wrongdoing, the death of a parent may make children blame themselves and feel responsible and guilty. They may spend much time thinking and worrying about who God is and what God will do to them. A parent's death may also be seen as a parent's or God's way of punishing them personally. Worries about being abandoned are also common. Fears of separation, although less prominent than fears of mutilation, are still present in this age range.

Fortunately, few children at this age have parents who die. However, deaths of relatives, neighbors, and other acquaintances can be very distressing. Because death takes on a personal quality some children suffer greatly while others may simply be curious. Just as their bodies mature at different speeds, so also do their minds, and nowhere are such differences in maturity more noticeable than in this age range. The following examples serve to illustrate some of the concerns and curiosities of children.

Some Examples of How Death Has Affected Children Ages 5 to 9

George and Tommy were both 8 when George died. That night Tommy came with his parents to the funeral home. After a few moments Tommy approached George's coffin and began to talk to him, telling him about recent events and things he did not want George to forget. Tommy's parents were surprised, but they did not interrupt. The next day, just prior to George's funeral, Tommy returned to say his final goodbyes and to add in several items that he had left out from the day before.

In another situation William, age 8, went to the funeral home following the death of his 6½-year-old brother, Donald. When the opportunity arose, he asked the funeral director to open up the bottom of the casket so that he could make sure that his brother was wearing his jeans and that his body was intact. He then proceeded to prod Donald's body and ask why he did not breathe. He wanted to know whether or not Donald was hungry and asked for an exact description of the final moments of Donald's life. Once William's questions were answered he was much more content.

In other experiences we have found that children have included a dead child in their play, talked out loud with the child, and shared toys as if the dead child were present. At other times children have pictured what a child is doing in heaven and continued the type of fantasy used by very young children. This type of response is illustrated so well in the poem entitled "Heaven," written by Claire Mulholland after her daughter died from leukemia.

Has God made her better yet?
my son asked, when
is my sister coming back?

Is Heaven a very big house
with rooms for crowds of people?
Is it very far above the clouds?
Has she got a big bed there
and a cupboard for her toys?

Is she wearing her big blue shoes?
Why does she not get cold—
is it very warm in God's house?
Are there carpets on all the floors?
How did she get in? Where
are the doors?

I will get a ladder taller
than a house. I will lean it on a
cloud
and climb into the sky
and go and see her.*

In other cases sisters, in particular, have been very sad and lonely at the death of a brother or sister. They have talked about how heaven is a place for flowers, trees, and sunshine and how their sibling will be happy there. The beauty of heaven is pictured as a way of consoling themselves and assuring that the dead child is safe and well cared for.

Further Guidelines for Parents

In this age range children who encounter death need to be part of the family. When children are properly prepared beforehand

*C. Mulholland, *I'll Dance With the Rainbows*. (Glasgow: Partick Press, 1973) p. 13.

we have found that inclusion of children in wakes or funerals at age 7 or even sooner can be a positive experience. Children need to know what is ahead and be warned that the person is dead and not sleeping. Their curiosity should also be allowed to surface just as William's surfaced. When the comfort and support of a parent, parents, or grandparents is provided along with a willingness to answer questions a child can be much less frightened and more willing to explore the meaning of death.

When parents or brothers or sisters die the closeness of family members to children makes openness and emotional support all the more important. Children need to know what parents believe about death, its finality, continuance of life after death, and so on. They must be allowed to seek strength and reassurance from what parents believe regardless of the nature of such beliefs. It seems that those parents who receive support from religious belief may face both death and children's questions more easily. However, it is important to remember that whatever *you* believe is what counts, and you must be honest. If you think that added help can come from a religious person it is wise to seek it, but remember that your child looks to you for guidance and comfort.

AGES 10 TO 12

Most children by age 10 realize that everyone dies. Many think about their own death and about life after death. Death is usually seen as terrible, horrible, and surrounded by gloom. Pictures drawn by children of this age are very realistic, and dead people are shown to have closed eyes and mouths.

At age 11 children begin to use symbols of death in keeping with their growing ability to reason and think in abstract terms. One writer* has noted that drawings may contain broken hearts, tears, or bare trees as symbols of the lifelessness, loneliness, and sadness that death leaves in its wake. Worries about pain and suffering begin to appear as children begin to think about their own deaths. They gradually substitute fears of suffocation for mutilation anxiety. As a result concern about death includes the fear of being buried alive. Such thoughts may lead them to private worries about having their bodies eaten by worms or insects. As children reach age 12 death is seldom, if ever, pictured as a person. Instead death is pictured as blackness and is associated with sadness and evil.

*R. Lonetto, *Children's Conceptions of Death*. (New York: Springer, 1980) pp. 146-157.

In this preadolescent period children are at a midpoint or turning point in their development. Death becomes more abstract or spiritual. Death is personal, universal, and real. Anxiety reflects the beginnings of concerns of most adolescents and yet continues the fears of separation and mutilation from earlier years. These early fears, along with suffocation anxiety, never totally disappear. They are carried in varying degrees on through adolescence and into adulthood, where they remain static until situations in life reawaken them.

Mutual Help

Most often children of this age experience the death of a grandparent. Loss of these beloved family members can be extremely upsetting because the attachment has been so strong and the loss is felt so personally. Death is real, and the finality is felt at its strongest. Girls in this age range are prone to anxiety attacks as they worry about their own deaths, and extreme outbursts of sorrow are common. Consequently the emotional support given by parents and their willingness to discuss what is happening with their children is extremely important. With girls in particular the mutual caring relationship between granddaughter and surviving grandparent (usually grandmother) can be helpful. A mutual support system is established as both need to be comforted. Granddaughter may give her grandmother someone to care for. She reminds her that her granddaughter's generation will carry on. Grandmother can give her granddaughter the benefit of love and life experience. In return she receives the comfort and caring her granddaughter has to offer.

ADOLESCENCE

Although the problems of adolescence in relation to dying and bereavement are discussed in other chapters, it is worth mentioning here that all healthy adolescents have special concerns and needs related to death. As they search for independence and meaning in life adolescents are very concerned about their bodies. They want to be loved, accepted, and beautiful or handsome. They want to be different from their parents, and they use their friends as measures of their success or failure in family, school, and social life. Their emotions run hot and cold, so that sometimes they respond to even minor events with much more emotion than adults would expect.

Since death is involved with the destruction of life and body it is particularly threatening to most adolescents. The death of a relative or friend brings home the reality that life can be interrupted and the goals of adulthood may be destroyed or never reached. Death also means that the beauty, handsomeness, strength, and capabilities of a person's body are lost forever. When someone close to an adolescent dies the adolescent often wants to withdraw or deny the loss. If the person was young the reminder of the adolescent's own mortality may be too threatening and the adolescent just cannot cope. Rejection of adult funeral customs is part of this desire to avoid death. The public spectacle of sorrow goes against the wishes of most adolescents to mourn in private or to sort out what is happening with their friends. The exception may be when their friends are mourning as well. For instance, when one popular adolescent died his classmates came in large numbers to the funeral home and mourned openly. Many came to the funeral, and most stayed until it finished. A few remained in the anterooms, too upset or frightened to come in, and two girls almost became hysterical, so much so that they left the chapel crying uncontrollably. Many close friends of the boy came to the family home following the funeral, and several continued to call his mother or come to see her for many months following.

In the situation just described peers were sorting out their feelings together. They supported each other through this frightening and sorrowful experience. The reality that they too might die became very real, and for most the loss helped them to learn and to grow.

How Parents Can Help

For a brief period the natural gap between parent and teenager is apt to widen when a family member dies. Sorrowful adults are preoccupied with a loss that many adolescents do not want to face directly. They certainly do not want to "gape at a dead relative" and go through the whole ritual. Their ways are different, and they need time and understanding.

As parents, then, we are faced with a dilemma. How do we support teenagers yet still manage to give them the respect and freedom they need to mourn in their own way? The answer most likely lies in compromise. If the dead relative has been close and dearly loved, adolescents probably need to see the body and attend the funeral and burial. These events bring out the reality of death and parting and, in small doses, gently temper the denial that most adolescents need to use to protect themselves. Unless they wish to be present there is no real reason (other than those shaped by parents' worries about what others may think) for an adolescent to endure the visiting of relatives and friends to view the body. By the same token adolescents may need to escape from a houseful of relatives after the funeral or to be excused at times from lengthy shivas. Adolescents need room to breathe and to think, and their friends may be just as helpful to them at this time as they are at any other time. There is no set rule or pattern for parents to follow except that adolescents must not be left out. In fact, you may find that some are much more cooperative and understanding than you ever thought possible. Most adolescents are never really predictable.

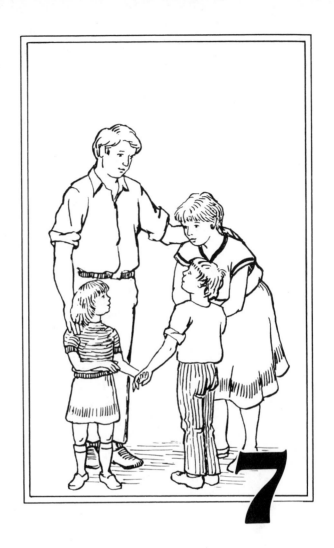

7

IF YOUR CHILD
IS DYING

FACING DEATH

Struggling with Reality

If tumors grow again and medicines no longer work to control them, or if leukemia can no longer be held in check by chemotherapy (and bone marrow transplantation is not possible), parents must face the fact that their children will probably die. Most have had warning that their children's bodies are not responding to the continued treatment. Despite this many simply want to deny that their children will die. They just don't have the strength or the courage to face the cold, hard reality. You may feel this way too. Like most parents you probably want to see your child achieve a great deal, to be better at what he or she does and be happier than you are. When reality threatens to ruin your hopes you may use several methods to consciously or unconsciously defend yourself from the tragedy. For example, you may be unable to deny what is ahead and become very angry or sad, much like at the beginning of the illness or at the first recurrence of cancer or leukemia. Wanting to believe that what is happening is a bad dream or feeling bitter or desperate are common ways of responding when life is threatened.

For most parents under stress it is perfectly normal for feelings to change from hour to hour or day to day. When you consider that such changes happen to everyone in your family, including your sick child, it is no wonder that it is sometimes hard to relate to or understand one another. When death is the final outcome of your child's illness you cannot help but go through a whole range of feelings that can be both useful and destructive. These are unsettling, and parents constantly struggle to keep a balance in their life and to control what is happening. This struggle also leads them to search for answers and to set goals that can be reached while their children are alive.

155

The Final Search for a Miracle

Several concerns arise for parents who learn that their children's lives are no longer being counted in years but in months, days, or even hours. The first is the need to be reassured that everything possible has been done. Parents must feel that the very best medical care has been given and that they can do nothing more for their children. The most striking examples of this come when parents explore whether or not they should seek other medical advice. Most often they wonder whether the doctors have done everything in their power. In desperation some parents seek out faith healers, looking for a miracle and hoping that something will save their children. Some search for miracle drugs or cures that may be offered in another country. Others latch on to remedies that are suddenly made public by the newspapers and appear to be the answer to everything. Most times the actions of families will be governed by their children's physicians' ability to completely explore every avenue of treatment. This faith and the trust that accompanies it usually grow through time.

Quite naturally, then, you may explore your own trust in the physicians who have treated your child. You may also ask whether searches for miracles are successful. To this we can only say that some parents have made decisions to travel great distances for another medical opinion only to find that their dying child suffers because of anxiety created by the trip, the extra fatigue that it brings, and the pain of additional tests. Some parents have taken the same type of tiring journey and gone into debt to buy a miracle drug that has added nothing but hurt for their child and debt for the family. We have also seen a child become sicker because a faith healer interpreted the appearance of a severe body rash as proof that leukemia was being drawn out of the body as part of the faith healer's cure. In fact a severe infection was out of control, and became worse, and because of delayed treatment the child became so sick that he could have easily died sooner than expected.

In our experience parents who have turned to faith healing or sought religious cures may have benefited from the comfort of prayer and the renewal of faith, but their children have still died.

To want to save your child is natural and normal. So also is the need and the desire to cling to hope. To act without thought and planning may, however, bring much emotional and physical pain as well as grief. Most parents need to keep hoping but also need to be realistic. They must continue to keep in mind the need for comfort in the remaining days of their children's lives. To find the balance between hoping, facing death realistically, and satisfying yourselves and your family that you have done all that you can is a challenge that many families have trouble meeting alone. Working with your child's physician and his or her team may save you much added strain and heartache.

Some Questions to Ask Yourself

There are several questions that may help you think about what you should do when your child is dying. You may ask yourself: Will a change now hurt my child or make him sicker? Will he or she suffer more? Will the pain and more sickness result in cure? What are the real outcomes of new or different treatments? Will these treatments interfere with medical care that is keeping the disease under control at present or keeping my child free of pain? If you are convinced that new approaches will not hurt your child, lead to bankruptcy, or interfere with medical care, will the fact that you are still trying to do something to cure your child make you or your partner feel better? All that we are suggesting is that you examine possible actions very carefully and look before you leap into action that may make you feel worse later on.

Setting Goals

Just as feelings change, so do goals for life. The struggle of continuous treatments and the original threat to their children's lives force many parents to gear down to a day-to-day existence. However, when a child is well some days are filled with hope for the future. When death is near such hope tends to vanish and families are challenged to get the most out of each day. As one father pointed out, "All my values have changed in these few short weeks; everything I valued before is now in second place." He kept his job, helped care for his other child at home, and even stayed at the hospital whenever he could. What he was able to give his son could not be measured in dollars and cents or trips to wonderful places, but could be measured in moments of happiness spent in play, comforting, and sharing himself with his dying child.

HOW PARENTS ARE AFFECTED

Worry about Their Survival and Rehearsing Death

When children are dying most parents have nightmares about their children's deaths or daydreams about how they will plan the funeral. For months many worry about how they themselves will survive. "Can I make it through?", "Will I break down?", "Am I strong enough to face the loss of my child?" are all common concerns expressed by parents. As the reality of death comes closer such worries become more intense. Rehearsing death and funerals by dreaming or daydreaming helps parents prepare for the reality ahead.

Although thinking about a dead child, a funeral, and a burial may be upsetting to some people, many parents have said that they need to have such thoughts. Such thinking and the accompanying feelings have helped them to face both the death of their child and the time after death.

Concern About Treatment, Time Remaining, and Pain

Treatment and Time Remaining. Just as parents worry about their own survival and their child's death they also worry about methods of treatment, the amount and quality of the time remaining, and the amount of suffering involved. Detailed answers to the first question can only be given by a child's physician. We have attempted to provide an overview of treatment methods in Chapters 1 and 3, and re-reading them may prove helpful to you. Obtaining answers about the length of time left in a child's life is usually more difficult. Often it is not until a child is within a few days or hours of death that a physician will even begin to estimate the amount of time remaining.

Pain. The third question is more easily dealt with here. Parents ask, "Will my child suffer?" "Can pain be controlled?" Parents hate to see any child suffer, especially their own. Three mothers who were waiting in the outpatient clinic for their children to be examined showed how much they cared about another child. They had been talking for a long time when a member of the clinic team approached. They immediately told him that they had just heard about the death of a boy who had attended the clinic recently. Foremost on their minds were the questions, "Did he suffer?", "Was he in any pain?", "Did he die in peace?" Fortunately, these mothers could be reassured that the child's death had been as they had hoped.

Recent developments have led physicians to pay greater attention to the need to control pain, and in some hospitals most children can be maintained free of pain and fully conscious until close to the actual time of their death. Some hospitals have also added palliative care programs, which remove the strain of trying to cure patients and substitute instead the goals of pain control and maintenance of the quality of life.

If your child has pain that is being controlled by medication it is worth knowing that most pain subsides for brief periods, even when doses of medication are small. This means that whether your child is at home or in the hospital, there will likely be times during the day or night when he may be alert or talkative. In instances when this has happened parents have been astounded at the speed of the change. For instance, 3-year-old Freddy almost died one day and the next morning was begging his mother to take him around the ward in his wagon. Bonnie, age 6, was in pain and dying at home in the morning and by afternoon was sitting up visiting with neighborhood friends. Such remissions from pain are common, offer respite at least briefly, and may provide some pleasant memories close to the end of a child's life.

In some instances there may be concern that children may become addicted while receiving regular doses of narcotics to control their pain. Medical authorities have pointed out that oral narcotics are not absorbed uniformly and that large doses may be necessary to achieve control. It must be stressed that pain management requires the expert guidance of a knowledgeable physician in order to be successful.

Concern About Where a Child Should Die and What Will Happen

Most parents wish to know where death should occur and what will actually take place. Should they take their children home and keep them there, or is it safer to rely on the hospital? "Will Jerry bleed to death?", "Will our child suffocate?", "Will he be awake?", "Will he know what's going on?" are all questions that parents ask repeatedly. They worry that they will not be able to care for or comfort their children at the time of death. They also worry that the actual death may be a horrible struggle.

Where Should Death Occur?

Death at Home. Today increasing numbers of physicians realize that death at home may be more comforting than death in the hospital. There are advantages to caring for the dying in either place. Death at home offers children familiar objects and the comfort of their own room. Access to pets, playmates, brothers and sisters, and the back yard means that the atmosphere is more relaxed than in the hospital. It has been suggested that death at home is easier for parents and that families adjust better after death when care has been given as a continuation of family life. The fact that dying children are not isolated and that death occurs naturally helps everyone take part in their care. Usually pain control is easier too, because children are less anxious at home and it is easier to keep their minds off their illness.

Death at home does require that certain safeguards be provided for parents. For instance, they must have easy access to medical care. Sometimes family doctors will provide whatever is required. Sometimes the cancer treatment center has a "24-Hour Hot Line." When a child dies at home a doctor must pronounce the child dead; therefore it is essential that arrangements be made in advance with the family physician to come to the home at the time of death. Otherwise the child's body may need to be taken to a hospital to be pronounced dead. Arrangements with the family doctor can be made either by the cancer treatment team or by the family directly.

A home care program with visiting nurses and social workers may be offered by the hospital or the community. Home care staff, whether hospital or community-based, can be of great value, not just because they change dressings, but because they can offer opinions about what's happening to a dying child, help mothers provide nursing care, and give families the emotional support that comes from regular contact and reassurance. In areas where home care services do not exist, this kind of help may be available on a limited basis through public health nursing programs or from special services provided by the community.

Death in the Hospital. Death at home may not be possible for some children. Family problems, overcrowding or other housing difficulties, extreme medical deterioration, and the need for special procedures are all reasons why it may be necessary to have a child die in the hospital. However, the most frequent problem is that parents are frightened. They worry about their inability to manage whatever happens. Their commonest concern is that their child will suffocate or bleed to death. Most parents have never experienced death before and don't know who will help them. Some also want to protect their other children from seeing their sick child suffer and deteriorate. It is hard enough for the parents themselves, let alone for the rest of the family.

Although we discussed the problems of single parents elsewhere, it is worth mentioning here that many will have difficulty because care at home is a 24-hour venture. Around-the-clock care means no rest, no peace, and continued demands from an irritable and sick child. Under these circumstances keeping the family organized becomes almost impossible for a parent on his or her own.

When medical conditions require hospitalization for pain or disease control it may well be that the only way a child can be managed at home is for brief intervals, providing the child can travel. We have seen situations where even a short interlude at home makes a happy break from the monotony of the hospital.

We have experienced a variety of successes and failures on both fronts. For example, when 8-year-old Brenda was at home she felt the strain in the family. She suffered more there and wanted to be in the hospital. Another child, 10-year-old Anna, wanted to go home to see her animals. Once she had done so she was content to come back to the hospital to die. Louise, age 17, chose to remain in the hospital when she felt that being in her own room at home was too upsetting and disruptive for the rest of the family. Eight-year-old Larry, who wanted to continue to be part of baseball and school despite the fact that his leukemia was in advanced stages, stayed home to play baseball as long as he could. The day before he died he left the hospital temporarily to attend a class picnic. For him, being at the hospital meant that he was closer to his doctors than he would be in his small home community, which was 40 miles away. Being in the hospital also allowed his grandmother, who lived nearby, the chance to keep in close touch with him. She alternated with his parents, and her love and comfort played an important part in his care.

Which Is Best for You?

When you must consider what is best for you and your child it will be important to discuss the possibilities with your child's physicians. There is no clear-cut answer as to whether death at home or in the hospital is best. For some parents care in the hospital is reassuring because they know that their child is receiving the best of care. For others the hospital is an inconvenience and an imposition. They may have difficulty trusting hospital staff to provide adequate care or may feel that their child would be happier at home. Ask yourself how you can manage best, what your child thinks or feels, what care is really needed, and whether or not you are capable of giving it yourselves. In addition you should know what the doctor has to say. Does he or she think that care can only be given in the hospital? Do you have a family doctor who can and will care for your child at any time of the night or day? Have you been told whether or not any type of home care program is available? Do you know how much it will cost?

Weighing these factors and reading the next section may give you a clearer picture of what will make the most sense for you, your child, and your family. Remember that there is no general rule. You should have a say in what happens, and you need the facts to help you make a sensible decision.

YOU AND YOUR PARTNER

The Strain of Terminal Care in the Hospital

Sharing in your child's care becomes increasingly important as death approaches. The strain of the threatened loss and the fact that children are often tired and irritable tests most marriages. We have already pointed out in earlier chapters how gaps in relationships can widen, especially when problems mount and feelings get in the way of communication. Common difficulties that may be present during terminal care include:

1. Problems related to money. Illness is costly and bills may pile up beyond reach very quickly.

2. Increases in emotional problems due to the long-term stress of illness.
3. Increased reliance on alcohol or drugs as a means to calm nerves or to blot out what is happening.
4. Disruptions in sexual relationships.

The burden of a dying child strains parents in two directions. First, they become fatigued. It is exhausting to keep going to the hospital and have little to do there but watch over a sick child. It is even more tiring to remain at the hospital for days on end. Although Mother's presence is desirable it can lead to a pattern where children become more and more demanding and mothers feel more and more guilty about leaving, even for short periods. Tired mothers have a problem because they believe that they are the only ones who can help their sick children. If mothers take over most aspects of their children's care and feel totally needed, both mothers and children benefit for a little while, but soon problems set in. Too often mothers and children begin to see nurses as being second-best. As one study pointed out, parents who smother their child with attention can create more problems than those who see both the need to be there and the need to spend some time away. Parents who can alternate with one another or with Grandmother help themselves and their children as well. A variety of family members who stay with the dying child at different times can relieve the monotony and the intense reliance on Mother. Mother can still be there when a child needs her most, but she needs a change, a respite, and a chance to see her husband and her other children too.

Once again, just as at the time of diagnosis, hospitalization for terminal care means changes in roles and relationships. Managing the household is often left to Dad and older children, whereas Mother is absent and sorely missed. Father, if he is lucky, may receive help from other children, relatives, or neighbors. However, little or no time is provided for opportunities for Mom and Dad to be alone so that they can support and care for each other or plan their daily lives together.

The Strain of Terminal Care at Home

When a child is dying at home the strain remains, but the whole family may share it. Some families will pull together; each person takes on new tasks and care is shared with brothers and sisters. Their contribution may come simply from talking, listening, or playing with their dying sibling. They can help to relieve boredom and provide diversion at times when a dying child needs a change from parents or other adults.

On the negative side, the dying child's need for 24-hour care means that regular living patterns are disrupted. For example, parents frequently move their sick children into the parents' room so that they will be able to hear or see them. Several parents have told us that they were worried that their children might die alone if left in their own rooms. The strain of listening and of watching over children means that sleep comes only in brief intervals, and parents gradually become more and more fatigued. Social lives and regular communication between husband and wife usually vanish. As one mother pointed out, her rest was an outing to the supermarket while Father cared for their daughter for a couple of hours. As children become sicker it becomes more difficult for parents, especially mothers, to entrust their care to anyone.

If the family can manage, care at home does offer parents a chance to relieve and help each other with the tasks of nursing a dying child. Parents have told us how much easier it is when they do not have to travel to the hospital and how much Mother's sharing in daily management of the household offers greater stability than when she is away. Nevertheless, the strain and monotony are present just as in the hospital. No matter how much parents love their children and want to care for them, there are times when love and patience wear thin.

When you are faced with this situation and you become tired and irritable it is important to remember that it is not a time to feel guilty; you are only human. In reality most parents do reach the end of their endurance at some point. This may be very hard for you to accept. The danger is that if both you and your partner are fatigued you may take out your frustrations on each other. The trick is to be able to know when either or both of you have reached the limit and have ways ready to remedy the problem. For instance, parents may send their partner out. When 2-year-old Carla was dying, her mother went out to play Bingo, swim, or visit with a neighbor at least two nights a week, while her father continued bowling on some alternate nights. Both said that they knew that regardless of what was happening each of them needed relief. Another family arranged to keep 8-year-old Andrea at home as long as they felt capable. When they became totally fatigued they contacted the hospital and she was readmitted for a few days. This plan gave the parents a change from 24-hour care and helped them to find time to sleep as well. Andrea also reacted to the stress of life at home and was much calmer in the hospital, slept better, and was prepared to go home again in a few days. Another family found that their health insurance allowed for private duty nursing. The employment of a nurse for the night shift made life easier for the whole family.

The amount of stress placed on the relationship between parents usually depends upon the time that is taken up in caring for their dying children. We have continued to be impressed with the resourcefulness of parents and their efforts to work together. Death at home seems the most acceptable way to follow when parents have a solid partnership complete with the ability to communicate, to share, and to care for each other. If such a partnership is lacking, bringing the added strain of a dying child into an already stressful situation will usually make matters worse and everyone will suffer—especially the sick child.

When you are faced with the problem of whether or not to bring your child home to die, you and your partner should review the situation with your child's physicians to gain enough facts to help you make a decision. You may then find it worthwhile to ask the opinions of members of your immediate family. Often family decisions that are well thought out yield the best results. Careful planning can mean that much guilt, anguish, and grief can be avoided.

If You and Your Partner Cannot Cope

Most parents who cannot face the stress of their children's dying have recognized that problems existed long before the approach of death. Most have difficulties that have continued since diagnosis and become more serious at relapse. Such problems usually arise from difficulties in communication and in the parents' relationship. Most often parents are unable to care for and comfort each other. Instead they continually hurt each other and think only of themselves. A major example came from an upset mother who said "I am numb; all I can think about is my dying daughter, and all he (her husband) wants is sex, night after night." Because each parent reacts to stress and meets his or her needs differently at various points in a child's illness, it is hard for any marriage to run smoothly. This is especially true as pressure mounts and a child approaches death. In the example just mentioned the mother had no sexual feelings left and just could not react physically to sexual demands. She was fatigued and depressed. Father, on the other hand, used his sexual needs to release his pent-up frustration. Father's failure to care for his wife in other ways was the real root of the problem. He continually failed to support his wife's efforts to discipline the children, refused to help her care for their home, and left her with all of the responsibility for managing the family budget.

If you are faced with such problems it may not be too late to receive some professional help. Counselors can be of value and are usually part of your child's treatment team. However, they can only be helpful if you and your partner both want to work on the problem. We have found that it is common for short-term interruptions to occur both in parents' ability to care for each other and in their ability to continue sexual relationships. It is the constant bickering, long-term lack of caring, and continuous problems that can lead to separation and eventual divorce. Unfortunately, this may occur at a time when dying children and their siblings need both parents most and need them to be together.

RELATIVES AND FRIENDS

If your child has been ill for a long time you will most likely know who you can count on for help. As death comes closer it is usually the old stand-bys who will continue to be there to support and assist you. For some parents these will be family members, while others may find that friends are most helpful. Regardless of who they are, those who will help most will be able to face what is happening and continue to care about you, your child, and the rest of the family. Perhaps the most frustrating problem is not knowing why other friends and relatives avoid or abandon you. Many parents have been deeply hurt because their brothers or sisters have stopped all communication or have begun to behave strangely toward them for no apparent reason.

Perhaps it is worth mentioning that people are frightened by the possibility of death, just as they are frightened by the word *cancer*. Both are upsetting. Some persons who have been close to you may simply not be able to handle what is happening. They don't think that they can help or comfort you, so they make excuses not to come to the house or the hospital and are even afraid to telephone. They find many reasons to protect themselves from their fears and justify keeping their distance from you. When you understand why this happens you may wish to confront them. When some parents have done this their friends and relatives have changed and relationships have improved. Such confrontations helped these people realize that they were needed and really had much to offer.

As a rule those who wish to help don't see you and your problems as a burden and don't want you to feel guilty because you are imposing on them. Parents report that such friends, neighbors and relatives are their best listeners. They have patience and they treat the whole family like their very own. They are the ones who provide respite and relief for parents by keeping a dying child busy. They don't leave when the going gets rough. Most offer more than emotional support. It is the babysitting and child care, the help with meals and shopping, the driving, and the minor help around the house that all adds up. Surprisingly, such helpers may emerge from a variety of places. They may include neighbors; friends from the past; people at work; and members of church, social clubs, or parent groups as well as family on both sides. As one mother said, "I really didn't know that so many people we knew cared. I didn't know how helpful a neighbor could be."

GRANDPARENTS

A dying child creates a tremendous strain on grandparents, who may be poorly equipped to face such a loss. You may recall that the problems for grandparents were discussed briefly in Chapter 1. When death approaches difficulties sometimes increase.

If grandparents are well and can face what is happening they can be a tremendous support. Even if they have to come from a great distance they bring their life experiences and wisdom and, in most instances, help out greatly. They can provide emotional support to the whole family, relieve parents of the burden of care for a few hours at a time, and assist with many much-needed but routine tasks of household management. Sometimes the grandparents on one or both sides have helped pull a family together and given parents the added stability needed to make sound judgments, manage their daily lives, and face their children's deaths.

Unfortunately, grandparents may have other problems that prevent them from assisting. For some, physical illness and age have taken their toll so that they are not able to face the constant strain of their grandchildren's illnesses. Some-

times the continuous emotional strain means that grandparents become a burden for parents and unintentionally add
to a couple's problems. Some parents believe that they have to
keep the fact that their children are dying "secret" because of
the emotional and physical impact that such knowledge may
have on grandparents.

In the case of Larry, age 8, it was grandmother who was
able to talk to him about his disease and death. Her approach to
death as part of everyone's life comforted him and allowed him
to ask questions such as whether or not he could wear blue
jeans in heaven, whether they had school there, and whether he
could wait there for her and the rest of the family to join him. He
noted that great-grandmother had already died, so he could be
with her and keep her company until the rest of the family
came. In another situation it was the grandparents, and the
grandmother in particular, who helped a mother finally part
with the body of her dead daughter and then gradually accept
her loss.

At times the results of grandparents' involvement have
been much less positive. For instance, a young couple had to
keep one grandmother away from their son's hospital bed
because she would become so agitated. Her behavior was
unpredictable, and she would end up upsetting her grandson to
the point of tears.

If you are able to rely on your parents, you may count on
them to add much to the quality of life for the whole family
when times are rough. The fact that they are suffering both for
you and for your child is reason enough to consider carefully
how they can help. Helping, for grandparents, means being
needed. Helping enables them to reduce some of the guilt they
feel when their grandchildren die. Some grandparents have told
us that "even though it's crazy" they believed that it was
something they passed on that led to the development of the
disease and eventual death of their grandchild. They wondered
where the "family genes went wrong."

THE DYING CHILD:
HONESTY VERSUS SECRECY

Being Open and Honest

Over the years many parents have told us that the greatest difficulty for them was the problem of whether or not to tell their
children that they were dying. These parents have been

frightened that such knowledge would be very upsetting and would hurt their sons or daughters more than the illness itself. They felt incapable of explaining their beliefs about death and were frightened that they would expose their own uncertainty.

Let us examine several points that may help you consider what to tell your child. First, it is true that children with leukemia and certain types of cancer are more anxious than children without disease. Second, it is also true that the pattern of communication in the family is a major factor in determining how children will respond to illness and death. One researcher and his associates* have found that if parents communicate openly about the disease and treatment, then children face either good or bad news better than in families where parents are less honest or avoid discussing the disease. It has also been observed that close to the end of their lives dying children tend to distance themselves from their family and hospital staff. In families where parents have been open and honest this natural distancing is less marked and children tend to remain closer to parents, doctors, and nurses.

Death does not change the need to be open and honest with dying children and with brothers and sisters as well. We believe, however, that such openness and honesty is not simply a matter of saying that death is coming, but is instead a provision of knowledge, love, and security that reassures children. If parents can communicate both good and bad news in a way that reassures children that they won't be abandoned, the added security builds in the feeling that Mom and Dad will help, no matter what.

Along with the security comes the recognition that because parents are honest they are worthy of trust. When this trust and security have been present we have seen some remarkable examples of the ability of children to face death. For instance, Mary, age 11, became upset and cried when she was told that she would die. Shortly afterwards she decided that she would go home from the hospital to be with her pets as long as possible. She remained there until her physical condition became worse and then came back to the hospital quite willingly. Another child, Gloria, age 9, became much less irritable and much more cooperative when her parents were able to discuss

---

* J.J. Spinetta, D. Rigler, & M. Karon, "Anxiety in the Dying Child." *Pediatrics*, 1973, *52*, 841-845.

J.J. Spinneta, D. Rigler, & M. Karon, "Personal Space as a Measure of a Dying Child's Sense of Isolation." *Journal of Consulting and Clinical Psychology*, 1974, *42*, 751-756.

her approaching death with her. It was as if she found an inner peace to help her cope. Another child, Scott, age 6, was much less anxious when his mother told him that he was going to die and there would be no more needles and sickness. He was fed up with injections, nausea, and the strain of treatments. For several days in a row he lashed out at his parents. He tested his mother by swearing at her and acting in ways that annoyed her. Once he knew it would soon be over he relaxed.

Being Secretive

It is important to point out that not everyone believes that you should be honest with children. Parents receive lots of advice, and most of it comes from people who advise them to avoid telling the truth. In fact, no one can say what is right for every family. In some families discussion of feelings or problems is and always has been taboo. Silence for these families is a way of life. Discussions about illness, sexuality, and death are embarrassing or threatening for them. Some cultures forbid such discussion, and powerful leaders in the family enforce the fact that it is not acceptable to talk about how people feel or about what will happen to them. Other parents keep the silence because of their upbringing. They have never been taught how to behave when they encounter such direct honesty.

Unfortunately, dying children may suffer when parents are silent. They are left to find out for themselves what is happening, and sometimes their judgment is poor. As mentioned in earlier chapters, children, especially those ages 4 to 9 years, weave fantasy into their explanations, and this fantasy can add to their stress. Parents who keep secrets may actually add to the fantasy quite innocently. On the other hand, children often wish to have simple explanations to short, uncomplicated questions. They do not want a whole story all at once, but simply want to know what the adult thinks about what will happen. Sometimes, however, children are very accurate in their beliefs and thinking. In fact, their feelings or perceptions are so accurate that their knowledge almost borders on the supernatural. Parents who are inconsistent in communicating or keep secrets, then leave children open to both their own confusion and errors and to a sensing of their parents' anxiety. When parents are anxious children miss the reassurance that can be found in a trusting relationship. When they lie and hide things children may become mistrustful and behave in ways that upset adults.

Dying Children Know More Than Parents Think They Do

Perhaps the most striking example of children's knowledge about cancer and death came from a study of children with leukemia in a large U.S. hospital in the 1960s. Researchers there found that children ages 9 to 19 consistently knew about their illness, knew whether or not they were dying, and had extensive knowledge about other patients who had already died or were very ill. Parents were totally wrong in believing that their children were unaware of their disease and its complications. In our experience a good example of children's knowledge was illustrated by Morgan, age 7. He and his 8-year-old brother were in their bunk beds at night. Morgan knew that he had leukemia, but he had not been told directly that he was dying. His brother said to him, "Mommy told me a secret that I'm not allowed to tell you." Morgan said, "What? That I'm going to die?"

In another situation, Barry, age 11, had suffered through a relapse of his leukemia and was doing poorly. He was discouraged and wanted to give up on chemotherapy. It was not until after he had died quite suddenly that his parents realized that Barry had told his brother that he knew he was going to die. He told them that Barry had left his family's Christmas presents with a neighbor and had placed January birthday presents for his mother and sister in his clothes closet. He had wrapped everything in case he was not alive to give the presents to them in person.

In quite a different type of situation Eric, age 6, had traveled over the same 50 miles at least every 2 weeks for more than 2 years. Recently his leukemia had relapsed and he had been quite sick. The night before he died he insisted on returning to his own bed instead of sleeping on the cot in his parents' room where he had slept for several weeks. On the way into the treatment center the next morning he asked about everything he saw, almost as if he was worried that he would miss something. This was such a change from previous trips that his mother commented on it. Shortly after coming to the hospital Eric died. It was almost as if he had had a sixth sense that told him what was ahead.

This last example is not given to scare you. Eric was ill and he would have died within a short time. What is important is the recognition that children have more knowledge than most people believe. Children do think about what is going to happen to them, and they listen to what others around them have to say. When they become sicker they often recognize that they may not survive. Children are also very capable of reading the faces of hospital staff, their parents, and others. Whether they ask about dying or not will largely depend upon the response of parents, relatives, and hospital staff. If children sense that their parents are anxious they may wish to protect them. They avoid discussion that might upset their parents further. Some children, like Frank, age 11, may use some objects or observations to talk about death. For example, one evening when the ward was quiet Frank said to his favorite nurse, "See that goldfish there? (One of his two goldfish was floating upside down dead.) I'm going to be like him soon." When the nurse asked whether this upset him Frank said he worried about his mother because when children died mothers were loneliest and suffered most. Unfortunately, neither of Frank's parents could face what was happening, and Frank sought comfort from hospital staff instead. As one medical colleague stated, "After 20 years of dealing with over 400 families of children with cancer I have never seen any trouble arise from telling the truth and being open and honest. However, I have seen a great many problems when parents try to conceal the truth from their children."

Children Need Stability

Just as children need honesty and security they also need stability in their lives. Major changes in information or events in their world can be most upsetting. For instance, Monica, age 4, knew that her birthday was in the summer. When her parents asked whether she would live that long, her physicians said that she would likely die before then. When they heard this close relatives persuaded her parents to let Monica celebrate her birthday in March when she was well. Instead of being happy at her birthday party she became very upset and irritable. The family just couldn't understand. On the following day she continued to be angry and misbehaved. Gradually we learned that Monica was upset by the change and could not associate her birthday with the springtime. She seemed to sense that something was desperately wrong. In another situation a major religious event was held two years early for a 10-year-old boy. He sensed that the way the service was conducted was strange and asked why this event came so early for him. Unfortunately, his parents were not able to tell him. In fact, he died without being able to talk about what was really happening.

Only You Can Decide What Is Best

When you are faced with the situation you have to decide what you and your child need. No one can make decisions for you. The events described so far support our belief that honesty is the best policy. However, in another example, one mother told her 7-year-old daughter everything except the fact that she was dying. The mother remained with her daughter and cared for her until the end. She felt she had done the right thing and that she would do the same thing all over again. Her daughter died peacefully and was continually comforted. Who could judge that the mother should have behaved differently?

Regardless of what you decide you should keep in mind that the older children are the more they tend to know and the quicker they learn. We firmly believe that when there is a great deal of trust between parents and children the children tend to do better. Being honest and truthful may make your child's death less lonely, especially when you and your child continually share in what is taking place.

BROTHERS AND SISTERS

Why They Become Upset

Brothers and sisters should not be excluded from a child's death. They have attachments to the dying child that are unlike that of any adult. They enjoy secrets, schemes, plans, and pipe dreams that exclude adults completely. Children play together, talk with each other, and protect one another continually. When a child becomes seriously ill and is dying the changes in a family are often frightening. Parents become more tense and preoccupied and frequently give more and more attention to the dying child. He or she looks different, is more irritable, and doesn't play in the same way as before.

Just as at diagnosis the family's problems in managing what has happened may mean that very young children feel cheated, left out, and rejected. Even being told that their brother or sister is very ill may not help, and they frequently resent the dying child's inability to play. They may act out, throw temper tantrums, have sore tummies, and cling to their parents. All of these behaviors are ways siblings have for telling their parents that their world is upset.

Older children too have similar feelings, and at times their behavior may change. Symptoms of illness, nightmares, and asking questions about death or about their brother's or sister's condition may all be part of their anxiety. Sometimes when they feel lonely and cheated anger is added to their anxiety as they struggle to make sense out of what is happening. Sometimes they are worried that they will get sick and die too. If they believe that they or their parents have in some way made their brother or sister ill, they may also become quite upset and their behavior may change. For instance, when 7-year-old Duncan's sister was dying, he behaved much better than before. In fact, he changed so much that his parents could hardly believe it. Duncan felt that his parents were to blame for making his sister sick, and his good behavior was his way of making certain that his parents did not make him sick as well.

Sometimes it is exceptionally difficult for parents to understand what is happening. Twelve-year-old Ben was upset by seeing his brother die. Ben was a good boy who did as he was told. Throughout his brother's illness he had been very helpful to his brother and to his mother also. However, as his brother became sicker Ben resented the attention his mother devoted to him. Unfortunately, he could not talk to her about it. Instead, late in the evening he began pounding his drums and singing at the top of his lungs in a manner that woke the neighbors. He knew that his behavior upset his mother greatly, and it served at least two purposes. First, he gained her attention. Second, he punished her for allowing his brother to become so sick and their household to be so upset.

There is no doubt that parents have trouble being fair to their other children. Siblings are often shunted from house to house to stay with relatives and neighbors and miss the organization of home life, especially if their brother or sister is dying in the hospital.

How You Can Help Your Other Children

When you are faced with the problem of keeping the family together and helping your children cope the following points are worth considering:

1. *Help them go on living.* When a child is dying parents may feel overwhelmed. Because they are so sad and preoccupied they may stop doing routine tasks that other children in the family miss. Brothers and sisters miss the presence of

Mother, the attention she gives, or the special time that either parent has devoted to helping with schoolwork, piano lessons, or sports. When parents are sad siblings may worry in private because they do not want to be an additional burden.

When you are faced with this emotional flooding you probably try to escape, at least briefly. It is hard to be strong all of the time. It is also hard to find relief, to smile, or to laugh. Your other children have the same problem. How can they be themselves when the rest of the family is upset? They still need to have their own time and find their own ways to escape. For many, this relief is found in sports, music, play, or just being alone for a while. Time for themselves allows them to sort out their feelings or rest their minds from the troubles of the family. You can be helpful if you can remember to continue to allow your other children the freedom to have this respite and to go on living their daily lives as normally as possible. They too have to face a frightening and trying time and are poorly prepared for the loss ahead.

2. *Learn positive ways to express your anger.* When parents grieve before death they may be angry and short-tempered. Parents who are angry can be very frightening indeed. When such anger is present most of the time, it is easy for healthy children to feel that they are responsible for the way that their parents are acting and feeling. This is especially true when parents misdirect their anger toward healthy children. Siblings are made to feel that they are trespassing and breaking into a relationship between their mother and/or father and their dying brother or sister. They then feel that they are a burden, that they create problems and make trivial demands at a time when a parent's attention is needed much more somewhere else.

At times parents may direct anger at the dying child as well. In weaker moments parents sometimes become extremely resentful toward this child who has upset their lives, is making continuous and unreasonable demands, and is taking so long to die. Parents who have felt this way have been shocked at themselves and have felt very guilty.

Bearing the brunt of a parent's anger gives children the message that they are to blame. Children who mistakenly feel responsible for their brother's or sister's illness can easily have these feelings of responsibility reinforced. It is no wonder, then, that some feel guilty and rejected. In extreme

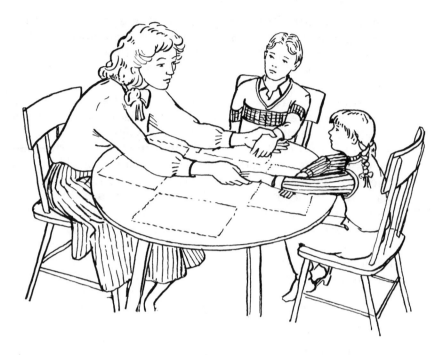

cases this can lead to acting out or to intense feelings of
jealousy toward a dying brother or sister.

When you are angry it helps to know how to release your
feelings in an acceptable manner. If you are in control you
are much less apt to direct your anger at any of your children.
The building-in of a safety valve into your relationships with
your partner or friends will help. You need someone who will
be there on the spur of the moment—and someone who will
simply allow you to talk and express your angry feelings.

Along with your ability to manage your own feelings
must come a willingness to allow your children to speak with
you about their thoughts and feelings. Sometimes just the
simple fact that parents can tell children that they also feel
sad or angry that this illness has had to happen can be very
comforting. If you can do this it shows your other children
that you are willing to share your feelings, that it is all right
for them to be angry too, and that you don't blame them for
what is happening.

3. *Be aware of how guilt can affect your behavior.* The guilt
   parents feel about their children's deaths may be quite
   unreasonable. For some, from diagnosis on feelings of guilt
   have been maintained. They believe that they have caused
   the cancer or missed the signs and symptoms so that their

children were diagnosed late. In most instances these beliefs are false. However, it hurts when the idea remains fixed and the guilt wells up and remains inside.

When parents feel very guilty they behave differently, and their change in behavior can be upsetting and confusing to other children in the family. Parents who feel guilty often become very restrictive. They want to keep their sons or daughters close by—just in case. They do not want to be hurt again. They do not want to allow their other children to become ill or to die from an accident.

The restrictions imposed by guilty parents can be annoying and hard to understand. At a time when children need to be supported and trusted, they are "grounded." They are punished without doing anything wrong.

Guilt may also make parents protective in other ways. Some mothers become overly concerned with the health of their other children. Any sign or symptom of illness may be blown out of proportion, and other children are subjected to unnecessary blood tests and physical examinations.

Sometimes when a child is dying parents who feel guilty change family rules and regulations so much that their children lose direction. Guilt makes parents totally remove the disciplinary regulations and guidelines that all of the children in the family have lived by and respected. When this happens children have to check out the boundaries and attempt to reestablish some limits. How far can they go? Just how much can they get away with before Mom and Dad clamp down? Beneath the confusion are the children's feelings that parents just don't care anymore. School problems, hitting other children, swearing, and staying out beyond the usual bedtime hours are all ways we have seen that children have used to try to regain their parents' attention and find new limits.

In earlier chapters we pointed out the need for you to maintain limits, particularly following hospitalization and during intense treatment. Now with your child dying the need for order is even more important. Sometimes it is worthwhile, at least temporarily, to turn over some authority to others so that boundaries and the security that accompanies them remain. For instance, if Mother is away from the home and Father is there only in the evening or at intervals, continuance of order may be maintained by transferring authority to a grandparent or neighbor. Even if their rules are not exactly like yours they are better than no rules at all. Both of you can still pay attention to your other children's school performance or play activities even if you do so briefly. Such attention will reassure your other children that you are still interested in them and that you care. If all of your family is at home and your dying child remains as part of the household attention to discipline will likely be easier, especially if you and your partner still remain at least partially involved in the lives of your other children.

In each of the three points discussed you maintain a central role. Even when your child is dying you are the 24-hour-a-day, 7-day-a-week parent to all of your children, no matter what. To feel angry, sad, and guilty is normal and necessary. If you didn't have these feelings you would be unusual, to say the least. You would also be quite ill-prepared for the death when it happens. You and your partner's ability to manage and to support each other emotionally are crucial factors that enable the whole family to live with the tragedy. Our belief is that knowing about what happens and why you behave as you do can assist you in recognizing how to help your other children. If, however, you cannot manage or problems grow so that they are totally beyond your control, do not hesitate to ask for help. In most centers cancer treatment teams have counselors readily available to them, and parent groups also offer opportunities for sharing of common experiences.

TREATMENT: FOR CURE OR FOR COMFORT?

Why Do Goals for Treatment Change?

When death is close treatment must change. Most dying children can no longer tolerate the strong doses of medication given to cure cancer. Treatment must be directed toward comfort rather than cure, or in medical language, treatment must be palliative rather than curative.

There are a number of reasons why cure must be abandoned. Sometimes it is simply that medications are no longer effective. For example, in leukemia strong drugs may stop being effective and cells multiply too quickly. The drugs that remain can not be expected to provide a cure. Sometimes when tumors re-grow radiation cannot be given to the same area again. Drugs do not work, and cancer spreads beyond control.

In some cases this turning point is expected. Parents have been warned at the time of relapse that it might or would likely happen. In other cases the change creates a new crisis, one that parents desperately wanted to deny or avoid. Many see this turning point as a time of giving up. It is a time when hope changes from a wish for a long life for a sick child to a desire for a short, pain-controlled period of terminal care for a dying child. For many parents it is a time of realization that 6 or 8 good weeks may be better than 12 or 14 weeks of suffering through agonizing treatments. For some, additional preparation is needed. A brief but final search to be sure that everything possible has been done may be in order. Time may also be needed to get rid of anger. Perhaps reinvestment in religious beliefs will also provide some added comfort.

If there is advance warning of the need to change direction in treatment the trusting relationship between physician, parent, and child can help the change take place smoothly. Emphasis on the quality of life becomes a common goal for all. A physician should determine the direction of medical treatment within new boundaries of suitable care for your child and discuss it with you.

Your Child Should Understand the Change

Since children are often very much aware of their treatment program it is important to see that their questions are answered and that changes are understood. Max, age 11, emphasized this clearly. He had been very sick and was doing poorly but was still being treated actively. During one hospitalization Max was not given his treatment because of low blood counts, and he was sent home from the hospital. No one really told him why he was going home, and his parents could not understand why he was so upset. Later he told clinic staff that he believed that because he had not been treated the doctors had given up on him and sent him home to die. At the time this was not true, and he suffered unnecessarily. A couple of months later he was able to accept the fact that active treatment had to be stopped because it was no longer working.

In our experience a number of children have been prepared to see treatment end so that they would no longer suffer. In fact, children may actually benefit from being able to choose (within limits) what should happen. For example, 2 or 3 days before Betty, age 9, died she was given a choice as to whether or not she wanted a blood transfusion. She knew that the transfusion would give her a few days improved health. However, she suffered terribly throughout the process. Her physician knew about her suffering and recognized that she hated needles and that she was in intense pain, so he offered the chance to refuse treatment. Another child, Joe, age 11, wanted a Bill of Rights for Children. He felt that he had suffered enough and wanted to stop treatment. He was content when it stopped and said that he feared death less than illness and treatment and really wanted to be left in peace.

From these examples you can see that ceasing active or curative treatment is a mixed blessing. For some, it can mean the end of painful procedures and at least a few remaining weeks in peace. Life may end more quickly, but what is left will be of better quality. For others, it is a dashing of hopes for survival complete with anger, fear, and anguish. For any parent, it is painful to lose a child, but as one parent said, "We have little choice, our child must suffer as little as possible, and that's all that matters now."

School, Play, and Your Child's Friends

As your child's condition deteriorates you will face new decisions about what he or she can do. These decisions are sometimes tied to medical concerns such as the chance of infection, fear of seizures (fits), concerns about fatigue, or worries about falls and bone breakage. Somehow you want to keep your child happy and also pay attention to what the doctor orders. As part of balancing between the two you are probably having to deal with your natural need to protect your child or to give in and let him have his own way. It is natural to want, as one mother put it, "to keep my sick boy (and my other two) in a glass jar on the coffee table, away from the rest of the world" or to feel that your child has been through so much that he should have the chance to enjoy what time he has left. As parents you will probably have to continue to recognize what your child can accomplish sensibly. How much can he tolerate? Will friends from school and the neighborhood be welcomed by him? Does he feel conspicuous or different, or believe that his appearance is so unsightly that he does not want to see anyone? Does he really miss his friends so much that he will welcome at least one or two of them?

Friends can mean that added change and pleasure are introduced at a time when a dying child needs it most. For example, friends can bring a renewal of interest in school or play. Sometimes they bring the well-wishes of other children in the class and provide some diversion that a child desperately needs. Because children tend to bounce back more quickly than adults, they have brief periods when they are free of pain and sadness. Most of the time you should allow your child to help determine what he can tolerate. However, there are times when you know that your child's sadness or suffering may be relieved by simply inviting another child to come over, even for a brief period of time.

When older children have allowed friends to visit in the hospital, small numbers of them have had a "cheering up" effect and have broken the monotony of hospital routine. However, if dying children have rejected their friends because of hair loss or other changes such as being bloated or thin, such visits may be too upsetting. On occasion older children have allowed only one close friend to see them, and this has been of great value because they have been able to share thoughts and feelings that they had previously been unable to share with either parents or staff.

YOUR JOB AND YOUR PARTNER

When children are dying the continued presence of at least one parent helps most of them. They are able to face pain, suffering, and the monotony of illness much better than if care is left totally to nurses or relatives. Just as at diagnosis and during treatment, you may have to make difficult choices. How do you choose between your child, your need to work, and the family's need for money? Most parents answer with their hearts, rather than with their bank books. The problem, then, is to choose who works—husband or wife—when they work, and for how long. Once again, it has usually been mothers who take a leave of absence or quit their jobs with the recognition that there will be lots of time to return to work after their children die.

When a child is dying a parent's presence is of value regardless of whether the child is in the hospital or at home. If a dying child is at home, parents have told us that it is very difficult when both of them are working because caring for the dying child usually means that parents get less sleep and become very fatigued. If one parent can continue to earn money so that the family can go on living, the other seems to manage reasonably well if the time is short. The breadwinner (usually the father) can help out at night and take time off work only when death is very near, in order to comfort the mother and the other members of the family. If possible, it is wise for the father to save a few vacation days as a means of relief when mourning continues after the child's death.

Although most parents manage well, occasionally major problems arise because one parent, most often the father, is too upset to work. Fathers who have stayed off work for this reason and who have avoided seeing their family physician or the doctor at work have often needed additional counseling to help them face the death of their child. In a few instances fathers have lost their jobs because they have failed to get such help and because they have not kept their employers informed about their problems.

RELIGION

Just as parents are influenced by race or culture, they are also influenced by religion or the lack of it in their lives. When people think of death many think of funerals and the involvement of a minister, priest, rabbi, or other clergyman. For some parents a renewal of faith can be a major support when they are facing the death of their child. The clergy can also be helpful. For example, our hospital chaplain helped one mother to understand her own feelings about death and life after death so that she could assist her dying child. At other times the clergy have remained close to families and comforted them as they faced death.

It seems to us that if religion has been part of a family's life in the past, then quite likely basic religious beliefs exist that may benefit them at the time of a child's death. For some, the presence of the clergy helps bring this faith forward when it is needed most. For others, it is the symbolism or ceremony of the church that is most reassuring and helpful. From our observations, people with some religious beliefs do seem to face death better. They seem to see more meaning in life and interpret the security they feel to their child.

When dying children have questions about heaven and life after death parents often ask what they should say. Should they tell them a make-believe story that they don't believe themselves? Or should they tell them exactly what they think, even if their beliefs present a very bleak picture? Most often when parents have told the truth children have been satisfied. They seem to want fairly short answers that reflect their parent's beliefs. At times parents have enlisted the aid of the clergy in such discussions, but the need for this has usually depended upon the anxiety of the parents rather than the needs of the children.

WAYS YOU CAN HELP YOUR DYING CHILD

When children are dying most parents feel helpless. They often find that it is a difficult and tedious process to be with their children constantly, and they seem to benefit from assisting in nursing care. In our experience in the hospital, parents who help out and still allow the nurses and physicians to do their jobs have usually been welcomed. This is especially true if parents are sensitive to the problems of hospital staff and share in jobs that the nursing staff have limited time to do. Some of these tasks are as follows:

1. *Mouth care.* Dying persons almost always have problems with dry, parched lips and mouths. Material cakes on the lips and tongue and requires removal several times per day with glycerine or some similar substance. When children are unable to drink or eat it is also necessary to rinse their mouths, perhaps by using a syringe. Special mouthwashes are available on many children's wards, and parents can be most helpful in seeing that such care is given regularly. The benefits offered include not only comfort to the dying child but also a reduction in the number of mouth and lip infections.

2. *Feeding.* Sometimes when children are small and nasal-gastric (nose to stomach) tubes are inserted, liquid formula or other fluids can be fed on a regular basis. The establishment of a routine feeding schedule and feeding by syringe can be time-consuming for hospital staff and a very worthwhile task for Mom or Dad.

3. *Comforting by massage, backrubs, and regular turning.* The problem of pressure sores created by contact between the skin and bed sheets occurs when bed patients are unable to move. Some problems have been reduced by air-flow mattresses and other nursing care aids. However, attention to the skin is still important, and gentle massages and backrubs are sometimes neglected when hospital staff are pressed for time. Parents who can offer such care every 2 or 3 hours not only help staff but soothe and comfort their children as well. This is especially true for children whose bodies are wasting away or whose pain is constant. A gentle backrub can also be a means of helping a child drift off to sleep.

4. *Providing diversion.* Perhaps the greatest contribution made by parents is helping to keep a child occupied.

Reading, card games, stories, and puzzles can all help break the monotony when children are well enough to participate. Although hospitals often have child life staff who help children each day in the hospital, there is never enough time for regular diversion or play. Parents fill the gap well. Even though such activities are boring and tiring, the contribution to a child's well-being is tremendous.

As well as the need to play, children need to remain in contact with the ward and the rest of the hospital. Time after time we have seen children who are close to death demand to be pulled in a wagon round and round the ward. It is as if the motion helps and being with others means that the child remains involved with the world. They don't want to miss anything. Although this is a tiring process for parents, it comforts the child and is a task for which hospital staff seldom have time.

5. *Observing.* Unfortunately, hospitals are frequently short of staff. Children who receive intravenous (IV) feedings must be watched, and sometimes staff are unable to refill the bottle as soon as they should. When no warning mechanisms are built into the intravenous system parents can be most helpful in letting staff know when their attention is required.

   Other types of observations that may be helpful to nursing staff include noticing major changes in breathing patterns, skin coloring, degrees of restlessness, amount of urinary output, and so on. Sometimes mothers, in particular, are first to notice even the most minor changes in their child's behavior and appearance.

6. *Protecting.* Although hospital staff may not appreciate this role for parents, it can be very important, especially if parents know that the role of protector should not be overplayed. Perhaps protecting is most necessary in the last 2 or 3 days of life. We recall one mother who stood at the foot of her dying child's bed and told the blood technician that she was not to touch her son. She would allow no more procedures. The mother repeated her verdict to the head resident, the child's nurse, and the cancer treatment physician. She felt that it was totally unreasonable to take more blood for tests and subject her child to more pain when he had only another day or so to live. Sometimes in large teaching hospitals efforts of resident doctors and the hospital staff's need to be efficient can cause them to miss the child's need for peace and comfort. Protecting a child can simply mean that you ask that only the minimum of care be given in the final hours so that your child can die peacefully.

At any time during the final part of their children's lives parents should feel free to consider their children's needs for rest and privacy. Although requesting privacy and time to rest may be in conflict with the staff's interests, the time may come when parents are justified in making such requests. Reducing the numbers of staff involved may also be reasonable, since children tend to resent large numbers of people coming into their room to examine them. The most important fact to keep in mind is that such requests should be reasonable and worthwhile. Parents who help out and who make reasonable demands will be appreciated far more than those who are always demanding and who are never satisfied.

As you will recognize, these points have focused on care in the hospital. If your child is dying at home items 1 to 5 will be just as important as if your child were hospitalized. Item 6 may be less necessary, or at least easier. At home, it may be relatives rather than hospital staff who need to be controlled, and this may or may not be more easily accomplished.

AS THE END DRAWS NEAR

Many parents worry about facing the final moments of their children's lives. Unfortunately, no one can begin to predict how children will die. We can only say that some children begin to have more difficulty breathing and then lapse into a coma (become unconscious); their breathing becomes more rapid and shallow, and then it finally stops. Some children enter coma states several hours or days before death, gradually slip away, and die peacefully. Others may bleed internally or from the nose and then become comatose and die. Since at this stage most children are being cared for on a regular basis by physicians, most of the time death comes peacefully and children do not have a final outburst of pain or period of intense suffering. Some parents have found comfort in reading about the "life after life experiences" of adults who have been revived. The peacefulness that these people describe has helped to take away some of the uncertainty and anxiety about the actual time of death.

In our experience parents have worried that they would not be present at the time of their children's deaths. This has been especially true when they have had to leave the hospital for a while or have lived outside of the city. In some cases children have hung on to life until their parents came and final goodbyes were said. It is important for parents to be there, especially when children are conscious. Most times, if hospital staff know that children are very near death they will call the parents and try to have a staff member remain close by.

FINAL PREPARATION FOR DEATH

A week or so before death the following points are worth considering:

1. *Making funeral arrangements.* Many parents have found that it is worthwhile to finalize funeral arrangements ahead of time. It was easier to do this when they were less upset and better organized than at the time of their children's deaths. Most found that the funeral director was helpful, reassuring, and comforting. Most believed that they had done the right thing. You may feel the necessity to tie up such loose ends, and only you can make that decision.

2. *Honoring the dying child's need to complete "unfinished business."* Just as you have unfinished business to attend to, so also do most children. One boy, age 13, told his mother to pack up all of his books and take them home. His mother did so, and he died shortly thereafter. He needed to have the task completed when he wanted it, and he became relaxed once it was done. Another child, Bertha, age 7, hung on to life until a friend came back from vacation so that she could see her friend once more. After her friend visited, she died quietly. Other children have given away toys or sports equipment as final preparation to put their minds at ease.

3. *Knowing about the post-mortem request.* Parents have benefited from advance knowledge that in major teaching hospitals physicians will request permission to perform a post-mortem examination (autopsy) on their children's bodies. This is a surgical procedure that involves clipping small samples of tissue from various organs in the body. It is helpful to physicians because it allows them to learn more about how the disease or infection caused children's deaths. Sometimes the findings are sent to major research centers and become part of a large collection of knowledge about the effects of certain types of cancer on the body.

   We believe that it is better for parents to be informed ahead of time because they have a chance to think about giving permission. Parents who are warned are not faced with the shock of hearing the question from a person who may be totally new to the family—often a resident physician on night or weekend call—who is placed in the awkward position of requesting a post-mortem. If your child is dying you can expect that such a request will probably follow. You may wish to ask appropriate doctors who are treating your son or daughter more about what is involved.

4. *The "no resuscitation" policy.* Many hospitals today allow doctors to write orders that state that dying persons should not be resuscitated (revived). It simply means that when death is inevitable heroic measures are avoided. No cardiac arrest procedures are followed, and the person is allowed to die naturally. When cancer is advanced and your child is dying, your physician may recommend that such an order would be helpful. Most parents do not want a child to be revived unnecessarily, so most accept the fact that resuscitation should be avoided under such circumstances.

THE FINAL MOMENTS AND THE TIME IMMEDIATELY AFTER DEATH

When the end comes you should be allowed to be with your child. Unless your child dies suddenly there is no reason why you should not be there, unless you choose not to be. The comfort you may be able to offer may help your child die in peace.

Once a child dies hospitals will vary in what they expect you to do. It is quite reasonable to remain with your child's body for a period of time, and most children's wards allow this. Many hospitals will also allow you to remain nearby while nurses remove tubing, prepare the body, and straighten the room. You should be under no pressure to leave quickly. Unless culture dictates otherwise, many families have found that this time is important and helpful and that it brings a much-needed sense of finality to them.

Leaving the hospital after their children's death has been described by most parents as a very empty experience. The most difficult part has been leaving with all of their children's belongings but without their children. Most parents who have had some warning that death is coming tell us that no matter how prepared they were for the actual death, they have been shocked. Some parents who have grieved for their children before death may experience a sudden feeling of relief when their children die. This is a good thing, although it may puzzle them or the people around them. Death brings the end to pain and suffering and means peace for their children. It also means that they no longer have to suffer the agony of seeing their children irritable, upset, and sick, and it means an end to trying to comfort their sons or daughters in what has sometimes been an impossible situation.

Because we believe adolescents are special, we have chosen to add a section on dying adolescents. This is followed by a section on single parents that ends the chapter. If your child dies the next chapter about the effects of grief on you and your family has much to offer and provides help that should be worthwhile, especially in the year ahead.

THE DYING ADOLESCENT

The Threat of Being Abandoned by Friends

For adolescents, the thought of dying threatens plans, hopes, and dreams. It is devastating for them to see their bodies deteriorate so that they no longer look like their friends. Many, from relapse on, become socially isolated. Being shut in or being hospitalized adds to their feelings of abandonment by their closest friends. When such feelings increase, teenagers reject their friends because they feel that they can no longer keep up, they are different, and others don't really care about them anymore.

Extremes in Behavior Are Common

Often a dying adolescent exhibits extremes of behavior. Sometimes boys become more active or aggressive and girls become more withdrawn and depressed. The point is that for adolescents the threat of the end of life can result in a continuous need to deny, to accept information only in small amounts, and to fight or run when threatened by such information or changes in their body.

The Struggle of One Dying Adolescent

Jeff, a 15-year-old who was dying from leukemia, showed us a number of examples of the behavior described above. Like many adolescents, Jeff grappled with his religious beliefs and found that his greatest comfort occurred at times when he was out in the woods alone. There he felt close to God and to nature and could forget the constant barrage of treatments that he faced every week. When he had relapsed for the third time and he realized his life was shortening he became extremely agitated. He accelerated his activities and moved throughout the hospital very rapidly, telling numerous staff that he had leukemia and that he might die. He sought comfort from hospital staff continually and called some of them at home in order to find added emotional support and recognition. When the social worker confronted him about his behavior and why he was acting as he was Jeff did not want to hear about it. He became angry and sought help elsewhere. When he was told that his chemotherapy had failed again, about 3 weeks before he died, he ran out of the clinic, and staff found him in tears in the back seat of his parents' car in the parking garage.

During the last few months it was apparent that Jeff had a need to set some goals and to accomplish some unfinished business. Part of the need for adolescents is to keep active, and setting goals is usually helpful. He wanted to join the Birdwatchers Society, and so he did. He also stayed in school and tried hard to finish his year. About 3 months before he died he planned a trip back to his home community, some 500 miles away. There he wanted to see his old friends and go back to his beloved forest. Once he had done this he seemed to be more at ease. As he neared death his ambitions gradually reduced, his goals became fewer, and those that remained related to living through each remaining day.

The great range of moods that Jeff experienced was typical of suffering adolescents. He shifted quickly and frequently from being happy, outgoing, and carefree to being somber, sulking, and irritable. Much depended upon whether he had to visit the hospital, whether symptoms of his disease were present, and whether he was allowed to remain at home in peace. Like most teenagers, he had problems relating to his parents. Attempts to narrow the relationship gap were only fleetingly successful. Father, as a key figure in the family, helped best with practical problems and was most comfortable relating to other family members around nonemotional issues. Unfortunately, Jeff needed help from his parents to cope with his feelings—on his own terms, of course, and only when he was ready. It was difficult for his parents to provide this. His tendency to be inconsistent in his relationships with most adults widened the gap between parents and son at a time when he really needed reassurance and encouragement. Fortunately, because of Jeff's nature he usually found help elsewhere. Some support came from his siblings, from hospital staff, and from a young people's religious group.

Friends Matter

For most adolescents the importance of peers continues right up to the end. Most dying adolescents will still tolerate the closeness of one or two friends as long as their friends will stick by them no matter what happens. As a result it is important for parents to recognize that these friends are very much a part of the adolescent's life and should seldom be excluded unless their son or daughter requests it.

Teens Need to Go On Living and to Control Their Lives

As Jeff's case so clearly illustrates, the greatest need for adolescents is to go on living and have the right to continue to control at least some aspects of their lives. Special foods, music, hobbies, access to the telephone, and the chance to be mobile are all extremely important. One teenager, for example, continued to run as long as possible; another played basketball; and yet another went fishing. Many show great acts of courage and fight back to beat cancer or accomplish a great deal in helping others. They show the same type of spirit as the late Terry Fox, Canada's courageous one-legged cross-country runner. As a young adult Terry had been treated for cancer and had his leg amputated. He wanted others to have the same chance for cure that he had had and so began on a cross-country run. With one leg he ran 26 miles per day or better to raise funds for cancer research. Part of the way through his run he relapsed, and the return of his cancer forced him to stop. The nation awoke to Terry's appeal, and over $20,000,000 was raised quickly. Terry's desire to complete his run continued, and he served as a tremendous inspiration to other young people with cancer until his death.

Adolescents want to have control, to fight back, and to help others. They will struggle and work together if they can really help each other. For example, in an adolescent group at our hospital both dying adolescents and those with much hope comforted each other and talked about feelings and concerns that they felt their parents and others would not understand. Following the death of two members the group continued and wanted to develop teaching materials that would help doctors and nurses understand the needs of young people with cancer.

As death nears and the struggle for control continues it may simply show up as an adolescent's right to limit access to his or her room, especially when in the hospital. For example, Ellen, age 17, had become pale and thin and had lost her hair. She wanted to withdraw from the world and have her privacy respected. She requested that several people be told to stop visiting because they upset her. Apart from her parents and siblings, others were allowed to visit only on her terms. As her condition became worse she continued to have at least some controls over her privacy. When she died she did so peacefully.

Dying Adolescents May Become Dependent or May Reject You

If you have a dying adolescent it is important for you to recognize that there are times when your son or daughter will behave as if he or she were much younger. Physical exhaustion, aggressive chemotherapy, surgery, and disease often make people more dependent, so that they rely on others for added emotional support and comfort. The shift to such dependence can be startling and upsetting. It can make you feel needed, but it also can increase your anxiety about your child's ability to cope with what is happening. On the other hand, there are times when adolescents become very independent and reject almost everyone. You may be a ready-made target for your teen's anger, or you may be pushed away at a time when your son or daughter wants to deny what is happening and "fight it off." When this happens you may feel helpless and rejected and uncertain as to what to do. As one parent put it, "What does Kim actually want from me?" Her question arose out of frustration and was repeated several times over when she was rebuffed by a suffering daughter. Other parents have been upset because teens confided in staff, friends, or other patients and excluded their parents. Attempts to comfort may be interpreted as being nosy, and more than one adolescent has angrily told his parents that his problems are "none of their business."

Points Worth Remembering

At such times it is worthwhile remembering that when your son or daughter is at his or her worst it is unwise to pass judgment or to change your behavior unless you have some professional help in doing so. More often than not your adolescent needs you and really wants you there but can't always show it. Physical comfort, hugs, diversion, and conversation may all be rejected at one time or another, but at least you are continuing to show that you love and care. Such behavior is not only restricted to mothers, but must come from fathers as well. Fathers are needed just as greatly, but they may feel even more awkward than mothers. Our belief is that as parents you often set the tone in relationships. If you are frightened about how to behave your children will be uncertain as well. Adolescents are no exception.

SOME SPECIFIC CONCERNS
FOR SINGLE PARENTS

Although most of this chapter has probably been helpful for you, you may have some special concerns and require special information if you are a single parent.

With Whom Can You Share the Responsibility?

You may have found that the problem of being alone has been a continuous burden throughout the illness. It is difficult to be on your own at diagnosis and at relapse because the threat of death is at the forefront. However, the experience may have given you the added strength and courage needed to face your child's death. The strain of continuous illness and fatigue usually takes priority. If a child is in the hospital the pressure of daily visiting and the provision of emotional support to the sick child often means that a single parent has little patience left to love and care for the remainder of the family. When a child is dying you will likely find that work is out of the question, and in most instances single parents find that their priority is trying to get through the days or weeks of terminal care. In our experience single parents are at a severe disadvantage if they use all of their emotional strength for their sick child, because they feel guilty that they are neglecting the others. If they try to care for their other children and cut down on hospital visits, they frequently feel that they are losing precious moments with a child who will not be there much longer. As a result, they feel equally guilty. The fact remains, however, that a sick child and siblings must be cared for regardless of how tired or distressed you feel.

If the child is at home you may find that the situation is easier because other children can be part of the daily care of your dying child. They can keep your child company, help the time pass, run errands for you, and carry out minor tasks under your supervision. The strain of travel to and from the hospital and the cost involved are removed. Your main problems center upon your personal comfort about having your child at home and whether or not you can receive relief from the constant strain. Can you, for example, obtain assistance at night, or are you on call 24 hours a day? Because parents worry about children dying alone and are fearful of how death will occur, they frequently sleep next to their child's bed. Without relief few single parents can survive the continuous interruptions in their sleeping patterns. The need for them to be constantly vigilant wears them out. When they become tired they become irritable, and everyone else in the family, including the dying child, becomes upset. Even in families where relatives are cooperative and helpful many single parents are reluctant to ask them to remain by a child's bed overnight, even when they need sleep themselves.

Another concern is whether or not you feel that medical support is adequate. Can you cope with whatever happens to your child physically? The type of support available varies from community to community. Most parents are frightened that death may be violent. Their children may hemorrhage to death or suffer from air hunger. If medical and nursing resources can come in each day and are only a telephone call away they may feel more secure. As a single parent you will likely worry about the burden of having total responsibility and may think that you cannot face the actual time of death alone. Without a partner you may find it hard to judge what is happening and to gauge when you need medical support. In some instances friends and relatives may be able to help. It is when they are not around and when you have no one in whom to confide that problems are most apt to increase beyond your control. If you feel that you are losing control you alone can decide how you can manage best and whether or not you need professional assistance.

How Much Should You Share
with Your Former Spouse?

Cooperation. When couples are separated or divorced many learn to work together and cooperate, sometimes behaving like old friends. When this has happened some former partners, usually husbands, have continued to see their children on a regular basis, so that when one child becomes ill their involvement continues. Sometimes this has enabled an estranged spouse to be very helpful. We have seen situations where a father has taken the remaining siblings for a few days to provide them with a change and to give their mother a much-needed break from bearing total responsibility. We have also seen fathers provide additional financial assistance to help with medical costs, transportation, and eventually funeral arrangements. In most instances this additional help has been welcomed, and mothers have felt a sense of relief. Even if they have not been able to confide in their former husbands, the fact that at least some help has been forthcoming and some responsibility has been shared does make a positive difference.

Conflict. Unfortunately, not all situations are so positive. When couples have been separated for a short period and emotional wounds have not healed it is hard for a single parent to share responsibility with someone he or she cannot trust. When this happens it is difficult for hospital staff. If a child is dying many staff feel that the separated or divorced parent has a right to know. Most staff feel that they should respond to this parent's questions about the child's medical condition and advise him or her of what to expect.

Ways to cope. We have used a variety of methods to help single parents deal with this problem. In our experience thus far most single parents have been mothers and have been reluctant to re-involve themselves other than superficially with a person who has made them suffer. Georgia, mother of Travis, age 5, had been separated from her husband, Aaron, for 6 months. Aaron had been drinking heavily. He was upset that Travis was in relapse, and he had been abusive to his wife. When treatment of Travis' leukemia was no longer effective and the disease went out of control Aaron wanted to be involved in his son's care. Georgia did not want to discuss anything with him or see him. The social worker and the nurse-practitioner helped both parties by arranging for the father to visit the hospital at a specific time each day when the mother went home for a short rest. Permission was given by the mother to keep the father advised about Travis' condition, and in return, the father was not to contact the mother in any way. For 3 weeks this arrangement worked reasonably well, except for one instance when Aaron was drunk and had to be asked to leave the hospital. When Travis' condition deteriorated so badly that death was only hours away, Georgia allowed Aaron to be with her at their child's bedside, and Travis died in Aaron's arms.

In another situation Bill, a father with strong religious beliefs, continually upset his former wife, Shelley, even though they had been apart for many years. If he visited occasionally from another city where he lived she would have as little as possible to do with him. As a single parent she resented the fact that he had virtually abandoned his children for most of their lives. When her son was hospitalized with a malignant tumor Shelley made certain that Bill was advised, and shortly thereafter he visited. Later, as hospitalization time increased and his son's medical condition became worse, Bill visited again. Unfortunately, Shelley was present and the situation distressed her greatly. At her request the social worker intervened and discussed the father's concerns and feelings with him. Appropriate medical information was obtained for him, and it was decided that it would be the hospital staff who would advise him if his son's condition deteriorated further. After this he left the hospital quietly. When his son was near death he was notified, and he later attended the funeral.

In both of these situations the children were hospitalized. This was easier for the mothers, not only because the children were so ill, but because the fathers could visit at separate times and hospital staff could help negotiate exchanges of information and the organization of visiting. If care had been given at home interaction between the mother and her former husband may have been much more difficult. If you are faced with an unhappy relationship with your former spouse you may find the following questions helpful in planning your approach to allowing your spouse to visit and receive appropriate information about your dying child.

1. How involved was your spouse before your child's illness became terminal? Have visits usually been upsetting or welcomed by your son or daughter?

2. Has your former spouse asked to be advised about your child's medical condition? Do you feel that he or she should know?

3. Have the hospital staff asked you for guidance about how much information to provide if your former spouse asks for it?

4. Do you need help in providing information or in organizing separate visiting?

5. Can you care for your child at home? If so, are you prepared to allow your former spouse to visit?

6. Can you accept any help financially or personally from your former partner if it is offered?

In some states there may be laws governing the amount of information that must be provided to a parent who lives apart from the family. Laws, however, can be very impersonal, and sometimes it is helpful if you make such decisions based on your knowledge about what your child needs or wants. Such decisions can also take into account your former spouse's feelings, and if you actually try to put yourself in his or her situation you may feel less angry. As one father said, "I know I have neglected my children. . . . I know I love them. . . . I know I can never make up for lost time. . . . I feel so guilty." When his son was dying he felt he had to tell his son these things, and his guilt compelled him to do so.

On the other hand you may find that your child does not want to see his former parent, that such visits hurt everyone, that you must be firm in protecting your child, and that the law supports your decision. Once again you must bear the responsibility at a time when you may have difficulty making such decisions alone.

Coping with Telling Your Child That He or She Is Dying

Although this topic has been dealt with in some detail earlier in this chapter, it is worth mentioning that single parents may have more problems than those who have partners. Bearing the total responsibility in the face of death is extremely frightening. In Chapter 2 it was suggested that if you confide too much in your children you may overburden them and increase their anxiety. When it comes to dying some parents feel that children, particularly those over the age of 10, should know that their lives are coming to an end.

When parents are faced with the problem of telling children that they are dying there are some personal dilemmas such as religious beliefs that sometimes make it hard for them.

For instance, one mother who was angry with God and very uncertain about what she believed was frightened that her son would ask her whether he was dying. She was worried that she had no answers for him if he asked about what she believed would happen to him after death. Her uncertainty was only part of the problem. She was afraid to face her child alone and was continuing her tendency to keep the family communication system closed. In reality, she had managed her family very well by controlling the information flow and governing the feelings that were allowed to surface. It is easy to say that her behavior probably suggested to her son that raising the matter of the likelihood of his death was forbidden. The practical problem was that she had to face her responsibility in the way that she knew best and use methods to cope that she had learned through past experience.

This mother attempted to seek answers for herself so she could become more open with her child. In an effort to be more helpful to her son she sought professional help for dealing with religious issues as well as coping with her own feelings.

Sometimes when patterns of behavior have continued for long periods they are difficult to change. Trying to find new and better ways of relating to a child when death is near can be very challenging. Even if you cannot discuss a child's feelings yourself and allow him or her to ask simple questions about the future, you may be able to find others who can help you with this. In some instances in our hospital, when child life staff together with the social worker and nursing staff have been able to offer this type of assistance, single parent and child have been brought closer together.

Your Vulnerability

As a single parent you have the problem of being susceptible to pressure from others. For instance, grandparents on either side of the family may be unwilling to accept the fact that medication will no longer control your child's cancer. They may insist that your child be seen at other centers even though his or her medical condition is deteriorating. When this arises single parents are placed under tremendous pressure. How can you be firm and unyielding when grandparents push so hard? As a parent you may have to be brutally frank in order to protect your child. If you know that nothing more can be done and that taking a dying child to another center will have no positive effect on his or her medical condition, you will have to find the strength to say so. After all, you have the sole responsibility, and despite the pitfalls you also have the power to control what others do to your child. You can stand your ground even if it means hard feelings. Parents who have done this have usually found that relatives not only renewed their respect for them but also began to see the wisdom in their behavior.

Your vulnerability can also be a problem when you must face the world outside of the hospital and your family. For instance, if your child is near death and you choose to make funeral arrangements prior to the actual event, you may find the process to be extremely distressful. Selecting a casket and making appropriate funeral plans is not usually part of the experience of young parents. You may feel that you must do the best for your child and may feel obligated to spend beyond your means. Fortunately, the selection of caskets seems to be more limited with children, and thus one major expense can be controlled. However, expenditures for the use of the funeral home, transportation, and arrangements for burial can be areas where overspending may easily occur. Single parents have suggested that they have benefited from having a friend or their own mother or father with them when making such plans. In most instances they have also found that the funeral director has been helpful in matching funeral plans to the family's finances.

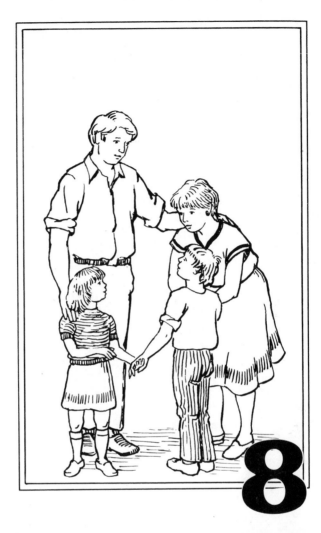

8

AFTER DEATH: HOW FAMILIES SURVIVE THROUGH GRIEF AND MOURNING

THE REALITY OF DEATH

The death of your child is devastating. Your grief may be so intense that you do not understand what has happened to you. Grief engulfs a person with overwhelming distress and suffering. Such feelings may last for days, weeks, months, or perhaps years. You feel that life will never be the same again. You wonder how you can now live without your child. Your arms and your heart feel so empty. You may feel very alone. It may be hard to stop crying.

The effects of grief are personal. Some people tend to keep their feelings hidden while others prefer to talk and to express them openly. If you are able to talk, even though it is difficult and painful, it will help you to work through the intensity of your loss. The impact of grief is discussed in detail later on in this chapter.

What happened to Peter's family is an example of how grief affects each person differently. When 15-year-old Peter died the whole family was clustered around his bed. He had suffered from abdominal cancer and was very thin. In the last few hours his breathing became rapid and shallow. Although he died quite peacefully, the time just before the end was very frightening for his sisters, ages 11 and 13. After he died it was important for them to be with him and with other family members. They talked about how different he was when he was dead and how "he had shrunk and looked like an old man." Being together and sharing the experience gave them a chance to talk about the realities of death. They were able to touch their brother and to realize that he was no longer alive. They talked about what it meant to be dead, and afterwards they seemed to be less frightened.

Peter's brother Mark, age 19, on the other hand, had been very hopeful that Peter would live. He tended to avoid discussing Peter's illness and to look toward the future. For a brief period when death was near he became extremely angry. He was critical of the nurses and unwilling to talk. As Peter's condition became worse a hospital staff member phoned Peter's father, who lived in another city, to let him know that his son was dying. His father phoned back to talk to Mark. At that point Mark said to the social worker, "He's really going to die?" Her reply was "Yes, it certainly looks like he's going to die within a very short time." The reality seemed to sink in. Shortly after Peter died Mark was alone with the social worker for a few minutes and said, "How come I don't feel anything? Why do I feel numb?"

IMMEDIATE REACTIONS TO DEATH

Numbness and Sadness

Death is frightening, and facing it can be overwhelming. Mark's numbness is one of the commonest feelings described by family members. The numbing effect is one means by which people are protected. It is nature's way of going slow and managing feelings that are extremely distressing. The relief that numbness provides can be short-lived, or it can last for days, weeks, or even months. In contrast, Peter's sisters felt their fear and sorrow throughout the final evening. They suffered openly, and their tears released some of their feelings of sadness. Their pain was more immediate and was not clouded by disbelief.

Anger and Denial

For Mark it was hard to face facts he wanted to avoid. His brother's death upset him. He did not want Peter to die. He did not want to think about it or face it or talk about it. Whoever was responsible for the disruption of his life and taking Peter away needed to be blamed. Mark's anger had to surface.

To deny death as he did is not unusual or strange. Denial is very common, and although it helps protect a person it can also make facing reality extremely difficult later on.

The reactions of Mark and his two sisters illustrate the importance of emotions such as anger and sadness and demonstrate types of behavior commonly seen when someone dies. Tearfulness, denial or avoidance, blaming as an attempt to focus anger, and delaying of emotional pain are all part of the picture.

As families leave the hospital or a child's body is removed from home, all of these elements of grief are present in varying degrees in family members.

The Time Immediately After Death

The emptiness of returning home without a child or the disbelief that it is all over hurts deeply. For some parents some of this void in their lives is filled with the hustle and bustle of advising friends and relatives of the death, contacting the funeral home, arranging for babysitters for other children, and preparing to have relatives stay over. The preparation often brings more people into the home with promises that they will assist and comfort the family. Their presence can be helpful and reassuring for some parents. For others, the numbness remains, and they proceed as if in a bad dream. The pressure of planning and organizing means that there is little time for parents to mourn, to be alone, to feel sad or cry, or to be comforted by each other. Too often parents are forced to put their own needs aside to comfort relatives and see that the household keeps operating until after the funeral is over and everyone leaves.

FUNERAL CUSTOMS

Faith and Funeral Customs

At few other times are you influenced as much by your cultural background, customs, and faith as when someone dies. Familiar traditions may provide you with some order and comfort at a time when your world is shaken. Although these may be reassuring for you, they may not be as easily understood or as comforting to others. They, too, are affected by their own backgrounds.

Religion can play a major role in funeral customs. For example, for those who are Jewish what is usually an immediate funeral and burial is followed by a Shiva. This time to mourn, when friends and relatives can be with the family, seems to be helpful. Custom dictates that parting with the dead person is quick but that the family is not abandoned.

For Roman Catholics and Protestants the events after death may or may not be helpful. Often the child is placed in an open casket in a funeral home where friends can view the body and visit the family. Some parents have told us that seeing their child's body again can be very distressing, while others have been comforted by the peacefulness. Those who are distressed tend to be upset by the appearance of the body—some are unhappy with distortions and some with the painted or made-up appearance. Those who want to deny death find that they are reminded of the illness and cannot bear to face the reality of seeing their child's body. Those who are comforted tend to see that their child is calm and feel reassured that the suffering has really ended.

For other faiths, the observation of specific customs and rituals can be comforting and reassuring because they stress the purpose of life and death. Most people, however, feel that much depends upon the person or persons who perform religious acts and ceremonies. Generally, clergy who know your family best are most comforting and reassuring. As one mother said, "Father J. is young, full of life, and very human. He knows us and cares about us, whereas Father C. is dull, goes by the book, and although he knows Mom and Dad he really doesn't know me or my husband or my children. It may hurt my parents, but we are going to have Father J. conduct the service for Tony."

Funeral Homes and Planning a Funeral

Most families today make use of funeral homes as a place to gather. Funeral homes vary greatly in their surroundings and in the ways their staff help families. Planning funerals and selecting the right casket and the right type of service are highly personal matters. Making choices about what is pleasing or right or required by society can be very hard indeed. Today most of us lack experience in making such choices, and occasionally parents' feelings may lead them to spend much more money than they can afford.

The nature of funerals can vary greatly. Some parents belong to memorial societies whose policy is to keep costs down and stress simplicity. For example, only the family may be able to view the body, embalming is limited, the body is held for a short time, and the casket is simply wood covered with cloth.

Other parents plan more elaborate funerals with decorated caskets, many flowers, viewing times of 2 or 3 days, and large processions to the graveside. Obviously, financial means and family needs have a bearing on what is appropriate. Most parents tell us that the funeral directors have been very helpful in sorting out what is needed and what families can actually afford. We have found that funeral directors are usually reassuring, well-organized, comforting, and offer the experience and security needed to help families through a very difficult time. Funeral directors tend to be highly devoted professional persons who are very sensitive to the needs and problems of families.

Should the Casket Be Open or Closed? The format of funeral plans, then, is largely a matter of personal choice. One of the decisions to be made is whether the casket should be open or closed. Some parents feel very strongly one way or the other and feel that they need to defend their decision to almost everyone. In our experience it seems that at least some viewing of the body is important. It seems to help family members to realize the finality of their child's death. For some parents it helps to see that their child is no longer living and confirms that the death was not just a bad dream.

The Time at the Funeral Home. Time spent at the funeral home has its purpose. People can drop in. They pay their respects and let you know that they care. Unfortunately, the process is tiring and comes at a time when you are most fatigued. For some parents it is an ordeal, for others it is a time to renew old acquaintances and gain emotional support from friends and relatives. Despite their wish to help you the probelm for most people is that they don't know what to say, and both visitors and families feel awkward. As one father put it, "I don't know what to say, I feel so out of place . . . so clumsy." When he recognized that the visitors were just as uncomfortable, he began to feel a bit better and his confidence was at least partially renewed. People genuinely mean well, and phrases such as "Sorry for your trouble," "I'm sorry this had to happen," and so on usually come from the heart. Attempts to comfort by saying "She looks so beautiful," "She is at peace now" are ways people try to reassure you that the ordeal has really ended.

When you understand how others feel you can probably take these awkward attempts to comfort in stride. Although comments may hurt because they remind you of your pain, suffering, and loss, in most instances you can accept them. However, some people do say things that hurt greatly even though they don't mean to be insensitive. We remember one mother who was told that it must have been easier for her because her son died after an illness—it certainly was better than being hit by a car! Another family was told "It was all for the best," and another was advised how lucky they had been to have had such a good girl; they could at least now live with her memory. It may help you to recognize that these attempts to comfort are made at times when people find the situation very frightening. They attempt to reduce their distress by trying to make what has happened seem less tragic. Their words are really directed toward reassuring themselves.

When people are clumsy and insensitive you may feel very hurt and very angry. You may choose to tell them so and feel that such confrontation will make them more sensitive. On the other hand, you may choose to "bite the bullet" and accept that they are trying their best. No one can make that choice for you.

Some people who come to the funeral home may avoid discussing your child completely. Most of the time they are frightened. They find that they just can't talk about the death or worry that you are unable to do so yourself. Sometimes you can help by raising the subject if you feel that they don't wish to. Other persons with similar difficulties may totally avoid the funeral home and the funeral. They may conveniently miss the notice or feel that they cannot face you, especially if they have avoided you for a long time. Others are just too upset to come because they have children of the same age. Later on you may find that these people still stay away, and, sadly, your friendship with them is never renewed.

Even when it involves some discomfort the clustering of friends and relatives can be a very positive and helpful experience. It can be a time of talking and reviewing both the happy and the painful events of your child's life—a review that you need to help you sort out what has happened.

The Funeral

The day of the funeral is usually a mournful and difficult time, depending on your faith. The weather may make a difference, and so does the way the service is conducted. Rainy, bleak, or cold days are very depressing and bring out the sadness in everyone. Bright days seem to be more reassuring and positive. Unfortunately, you have no control over the weather. However, you do have some choices in the way the funeral is conducted and the way the service is organized. When at least part of the service is personalized by the clergyman parents feel reassured and comforted. The trusting and caring that are offered and the rallying around of friends and church members can be helpful. Love, respect, and the purpose of life can all be brought forward during the service. Apart from the traditional religious ceremony, parents have found comfort in descriptions of their child and what was so wonderful and unique about him or her. No one can do this better than someone who cared about your child and knew about the contribution that he or she made to your family's life.

The Graveside

If your child is to be buried, then after the funeral service there is usually a brief ceremony at the graveside, where the casket is placed above an open grave. Some parents have told us that it is hard for them to leave the casket sitting there and that they have demanded that it be lowered. Sometimes the fact that caskets must be encased in concrete or metal means that actual burial is done by the cemetery staff later on. Parents who want an immediate burial often find that unless they have planned for it they are frustrated. If you wish an immediate burial, you may want to make your wishes known to your funeral director in advance.

Another problem relating to the grave is the cost of the headstone or grave marker. Knowing what is involved ahead of time is extremely important. For instance, today there are at least two common types of cemeteries. One is the traditional graveyard where some type of stone marker is required, and the other is the garden-like setting where graves are marked by metal plaques. Usually a flat fee is paid for maintaining the grave forever. A separate fee is paid for the headstone or marker. In our experience one father was very distressed to learn that he had to pay several hundred dollars extra after his child was buried in order to place a brass plaque on the grave. In most instances this information is conveyed by the funeral director ahead of time, and hard as it may be for you to ask when you are so upset, you must know exactly what you are paying for and what additional costs may follow.

Cremation

In recent years cremation has become more common. People who have had their children cremated have done so for several reasons. Some have firm convictions that too much land is being used for cemeteries and that they must help to relieve the problem. For others it is more economical, or it fits in with their religious convictions. Still others find the idea of burial in the ground quite revolting and unacceptable.

Like funerals and burials, cremation is strictly a matter of personal choice. Cynical persons have said that it is a way of getting things over and reducing reminders of death. In our experience such feelings are the exception rather than the rule. No matter how painful a death has been for parents, they usually want to remember their child and the special contribution that their son or daughter made to their family regardless of what has happened to the body.

If cremation is your choice, burial of the ashes does not necessarily follow but is optional, and many parents choose to do so. In the funeral home, after the service ends the casket is usually removed from the room to another part of the building and transported to a crematorium.

Gatherings After the Funeral

The final sharing of time together with friends and relatives at home or in a church hall can be the last show of support before everyone leaves you and your family alone. Inclusion of close friends and family is often customary. We have found that when hospital staff who have been helpful and supportive are included the experience has been excellent for both family and staff. This time is often one of relief after the funeral and is informal and friendly. It provides a chance for people to offer reassurances that they will not forget and that their feelings for you will remain.

FUNERALS AND YOUR REMAINING CHILDREN

What About Your Other Children at the Time of the Funeral?

For your remaining children the problem of grieving is as difficult as or more difficult than the actual death itself. Your other children are left with sad and sorrowful parents whose minds are almost totally occupied with the thoughts of loss of their dead child. The adult world at the time of death is often alien to a living child. Adult time is consumed by contacting relatives, planning the funeral period, and being sad.

When your other children are faced with the events of mourning it is hard for them to know where and how they fit. Death, funeral homes, and funerals are often confusing and frightening, and it is so easy for them to be left out. With this in mind, here are some thoughts that may be helpful:

1. Your remaining children are sad too. Much of what they think and feel will be related to their age. (See Chapter 6 on Children and Death.)

2. They may feel responsible for their brother's or sister's death because they believe that they had wished for their sibling's death at some point and that death actually followed because of their wishes. This is particularly true for children ages 6 to 8. At this age children have an interest in death and incorporate it into their fantasy life because they have much difficulty recognizing, understanding, or accepting the reality and finality of death. Even with older children who "should know better" the uncertainty of their role in death frequently creeps into their thinking. The "knowing better" has nothing to do with it, for with children, just as with adults, the mind does not always work in a practical and realistic way.

3. Children grieve differently than adults. Tears one minute and laughter the next are typical of child behavior. Fun, laughter, and play help them break away from the steady diet of grief provided by mourning parents. Children need this natural escape as a means of resting from their sorrow. Such behavior gives them a chance to recover and handle their next wave of feelings.

4. Just as you and your partner need comforting, so does your child. There is a need to fend off the loneliness of death in the family. Other children and relatives may provide brief breaks, but a lonely child is helped most by his parents, particularly his mother. This sounds like an impossible task. You are sad, grieving, and need to be comforted yourself, and yet you are asked to continue to give love and comfort to your family. As Schiff pointed out in *The Bereaved Parent**, Mother must try to move from being comforted to being comforter, even though this is extremely difficult to do.

*H. S. Schiff, *The Bereaved Parent*. (New York: Crown Publishers, 1977) p. 3–7, 82–85.

Should You Send Your Other Children Away?

Since remaining children are lonely, sending them away usually adds to their feelings of loneliness. Sometimes feelings of not being wanted or of being punished for having wished their brother or sister dead are increased by being sent away. Actually, attempts to protect them from the grisly aspects of death are frequently converted in their young minds to long-lasting feelings of rejection. If they remain with the family, other questions must be answered. Do you take children to the funeral home? Should they see their dead sibling? Should they go to the funeral? What do you tell them about death?

Should Your Children Go to the Funeral Home or the Funeral?

At the outset it is important to state that there are no easy or foolproof answers. When you are not sure what you should do with your other children regarding the funeral home and funeral, it may be best to listen to your children's wishes. Well-meaning but often ill-advised suggestions from people around you may be misleading. Letting your children be involved in this decision may help in their adjustment to the death of their sibling.

We have seen a variety of behaviors by parents, each of which seems to have merit. For instance, in one situation the family were all together at the funeral home. A back room was provided, and the three remaining children were there with friends and family while only one parent and a few relatives stayed with the casket. The social gathering was not threatening for the children. The parents took turns at the casket and spent time there with each child. They allowed the children to talk openly about what they saw and how they felt. In another situation the remaining brother, age 8, spent most of his time away from the funeral home, but his parents brought him down on his own. He asked many questions about his dead brother. He had time to touch and poke him and even made the funeral director open the bottom of the casket so that he could be certain that his brother's feet were still there. After having had this time to explore and understand, he seemed much more relaxed and content.

Some parents with very young children have excluded them from the funeral service but have taken them to the funeral home. One child, age 3, had great difficulty understanding the difference between death and sleeping. Another had trouble understanding why her brother had died, and another worried that she might get sick and die too. Despite these difficulties in understanding, most parents have said that it has been useful and necessary for them to discuss a sibling's death with the remaining children. When this can be done in very simple terms it seems to help and brings a child's thoughts out into the open. In one situation we found that a child was able to understand that her brother was so ill that he died, and then the child went on to make up her own explanation of where her brother was now. When discussion does take place, it should be reassuring. Sometimes finding out what children think can be helpful in forming simple, satisfactory explanations for their questions.

As a parent it is worth recognizing that you may have to give explanations over and over again to your child. Discussions should not finish but should always be open-ended. Explanations given at the time of death are beginnings for further discussions later on. Openness, honesty, and caring about them will help your children now and in the future, regardless of their ages.

One basic question remains: Should young children attend the funeral? What do you think? Will the funeral benefit or harm your children? Will it provide a feeling of family togetherness? Are you worried that you might fall apart emotionally and the experience will upset your children permanently? Some experts have suggested that attendance at funerals should only be considered for children who are at least 7 years old. This makes sense, but we must add that we have seen children ages 5 or 6 who have managed very well and who have seemed to suffer no immediate or long-lasting harm. We can add a question about the content of the funeral service to help you in your decision making. Are you having a lengthy Mass? It is worth remembering that very few young children can endure an hour-long ritual, whereas a 15-minute funeral service may be quite tolerable.

From a practical standpoint it is important that your children recognize that you are very sad and suffering just as much as they are. Just as at diagnosis, there is no reason to hide such feelings from most children. Children are perceptive and they sense when adults are sad. Many times we have seen 3- and 4-year-olds behave like much older children for brief periods when they want to cuddle their mothers and "make it all better." This display of caring and desire to share in sadness has brought families closer together.

Naturally customs tend to fit our adult world. Funerals, funeral homes, Shivas, wakes, and other rituals are for adults. As Schiff pointed out in her book, one of the greatest gaps felt by the teenagers in her experience was the fact that such customs were phony and meaningless to them. Even when deaths had occurred several years before, when the adolescents were children, their feelings were still the same. Children resented the adult customs and the way that these customs deprived them of quiet times with their parents—times that they felt they needed.

WHEN THE FUNERAL IS OVER

The Aftermath

Once the funeral is over and family and friends have left, or once the Shiva has ended, most parents feel mentally and physically exhausted. The ordeal is over, but the dream-like quality of the experience may remain. Some parents are so fatigued that they virtually collapse, while others are too wound up to do so. When you face this time, you have to try to make the change in your life acceptable.

Some people who have been on tranquilizers because the doctor or family feels that they must be calm and free of grief may sleep and grieve later on. Others at this point may need a mild sedative just to help them sleep and find some release from their intense fatigue. The constant use of tranquilizers or sedatives is usually inadvisable, since it just delays your reaction to grief. On the other hand, sedatives for a good night's sleep may be very helpful, since complete physical and emotional exhaustion can leave parents unable to cope with daily life. For still other parents, their energy has been spent in grief, and they are exhausted but at least temporarily at peace. Problems may occur with those who have behaved as "normal." These persons have not shed a tear, are seen as being strong, and are prepared to face the next day just as they faced the day before. We will discuss concerns about these persons in more detail later on in this chapter.

When funerals are over there are financial matters that must be completed, and for a while this may keep families—particularly fathers—busy. Sympathy cards and notifications of donations to charities trickle in. For some these wishes are comforting, while others feel that new hurts are felt with each card. One parent said "The cards keep dribbling in—it's not fair to keep hurting us over and over again. I wish people would understand that we need some peace now." Other minor business includes sending out information to government agencies and signing of legal documents—the housekeeping matters of dying.

Society's Expectations for Father

In society today many women work full- or part-time, but the main income in the family, especially when a child is ill, tends to be earned by Father. Because most mothers tend to be willing to care for their sick child and sometimes because their income is lower, they are the ones that most often take a leave of absence or quit work. As a result fathers are most often out of the home and one step removed from the emotional strain of the child's illness and death. Sometimes this distance makes fathers feel powerless, angry, or guilty. For some, being in control of their jobs and family is a sign of manhood, an ingrained expectation. They feel that they are responsible for protecting their wives and children. Although there is much more equality between husband and wife in households today, the weight of responsibility remains for many fathers. Along with this goes the problem that society still expects them to suffer in silence and to remain strong no matter what happens.

When fathers must be strong and not break down lest the family crumble, they have trouble grieving. They have difficulty before death because they often believe that they must cry and suffer alone or bury themselves in their work. One of our greatest problems has been in trying to help a father who runs away and avoids the hospital and his family in order to try to solve his problems and control his feelings on his own.

Ways Fathers React

At the time of death and immediately following we have seen a number of reactions. Fathers frequently become angry. Their anger is most easily directed toward physicians, and sometimes they do things they regret. Lashing out at wives or friends can be just as damaging. Sometimes these feelings are hidden, stored up, and they just burst forth. We believe that it helps fathers to talk about the death beforehand, face the reality of what's happening, and trust in someone in whom they can confide. This someone can be a wife, friend, relative, family doctor, or hospital staff member. Even then the feeling of having lost control and being cheated can mean that anger remains.

Besides being angry fathers may also feel helpless and be unable to function. In extreme cases we have seen fathers become so depressed or physically ill that they have stopped work and have had great difficulty returning. Sometimes this has been very hard on the family, especially financially.

The loss of a child signifies the loss of hopes and aspirations that can never be regained. For any bereaved adult or sibling the feelings of anger and sadness are normal, and these are discussed more fully in the next section. The main point here is that fathers are vulnerable and can become casualties when they lose a child. They have less chance to prepare and are often less willing to accept the reality of death. To make matters worse, society expects them to be a tower of strength, to avoid crying at funerals, and to return to work "fit as a fiddle" 3 or 4 days after the funeral.

The Problem for Mothers

It has been said that a mother suffers most when a child dies. Mothers bond to their children at the time of infancy, and separation by death later on means that part of them dies as well. Not only are mothers left with a void in their lives, but the hurting remains for months or years. Many people fail to recognize that mourning requires 1 or 2 years to complete and that there are a whole set of behaviors and feelings that must be passed through as a part of grief. Before parents can recover and reinvest themselves again in life they must sort through their memories and reexamine the time they had when their child was living. Although all members of a family must grieve, mothers often show their feelings most openly and are prone to suffering from a wider variety of emotional and physical problems. With this in mind, a complete review of grief reactions may be helpful.

GRIEF

The Impact of Grief

Grief has been described as the loss of a loved object, and a natural response is to pine and to search for it. People who are grieving struggle to keep themselves afloat emotionally. Anger, sadness, and guilt connected with the loved person are all mixed up together. Denial that death has taken place and longing for the lost person sometimes help to ease the pain. One psychiatrist has suggested that grief is much like a disease because its impact on the body may lead to development of medical problems. Those who grieve also suffer from loss of place. Their regular life changes, and their role in life shifts drastically. For example, Mother is no longer the parent of a sick child. She is the mother of a dead child, and people treat her differently. Often she is isolated, and people don't know what to say to her or whether or not to call. One mother said that she felt as if she were "tainted." Life at the hospital had finished, friends didn't know how to react, she was too upset to work, and apart from her husband no one wanted her. She felt imperfect—a failure.

Grieving Before Death

For anyone who has had advance warning of death, at least some grieving has begun. A mixture of anger, sadness, and anxiety have all been part of the preparation for the loss. A parent may move in and out of such feelings as they change hourly or daily. Many parents suffer from fatigue and recurrence of old ulcers and other physical problems. After death, the overwhelming impact of loss is felt in every aspect of family life. In a short time massive changes take place in the social, emotional, and physical life of most family members.

It is important to expect that grief will alter your life. It is the degree of alteration,however, that counts.

NORMAL GRIEF REACTIONS AND ASSOCIATED PROBLEMS

Emotions

Many parents say that it has been hard for them to believe what has happened. Some have described the feeling as dream-like, a sense of unreality. Some have wanted to remove themselves from others; they want to pull away and do not want to be touched. Others have become preoccupied with thoughts of their dead children. They cannot stop thinking about their sons or daughters and have an intense need to discuss their children's lives in great detail over and over again. They often visit their children's rooms and find that just being there is comforting. At times they may feel guilty because they believe that they did too little for their children. Some parents may also feel guilty that they ever wished that death would come to end their children's suffering. Occasionally parents continue to feel guilty because they believe that they missed the diagnosis or failed to protect their children in some other way. Many parents have found that they are angry, irritable, and even nasty, sometimes without knowing why they have such feelings.

Just as people move in and out of moods and experience ever-changing emotions before death, they do the same during mourning. As one mother said, "All of a sudden I hear a sound, and think of Timmy and start to cry." Another mother told us how dull, rainy days made it hard for her to get up because she wanted to stay in bed and weep. Another found that it helped just to have a neighbor come in for coffee and sit and listen to her reminisce about her daughter's life.

It is normal to suffer after a death. Painful feelings do not vanish overnight, and they are necessary because they allow you to express your hurt and disappointment. It is all right to feel cheated and angry and to want to remember what was good about your experience with your child. Remembering may hurt, but it also brings back happy and treasured moments that can never be totally erased.

How the Body May React

Along with emotional changes come changes in one's body, and of all the changes that happen these are the most surprising. We believe that one of the common oversights of family doctors is their failure to recognize some physical symptoms as part of grief reactions. First among these is the feeling of tightness in the throat and choking. This experience can be frightening and is very much related to tension. Such feelings tend to be more closely related to stress and fatigue than to the actual conscious remembering of a dead son or daughter. When a parent is frightened by these physical changes the problem can increase. Shortness of breath is another common reaction that shocks young adults. The reaction is similar to that of the tight throat, and it can be just as alarming.

When people are mourning they often feel "draggy" and sigh continually, seeming to be always tired and bored.

Sometimes feelings of emptiness and weak muscles are part of the physical reaction.

All of these symptoms are normal bodily responses to sadness. Many grieving parents experience at least some of them. If you feel different physically and recognize some of these reactions you should still discuss them with your doctor, but be sure to tell him or her about your experiences in the last few weeks or months.

Restlessness

Many bereaved parents have told us that they feel restless. They cannot concentrate or stay put in one place. One mother told us that when she could not stay in the house she wandered about the shopping malls. Another couldn't do any housework because she just wandered throughout the house aimlessly. Another said, "It is as if I am going through the motions. I just don't have my heart in anything anymore."

This reaction, like other physical and emotional changes, is closely linked to the depressive part of grief. Activities of everyday life become impossible, and people lose their ability to be self-starters. It may take prodding by a friend or neighbor to get anything done. This is especially true when it comes to doing housework or accomplishing a variety of other daily tasks.

This slowing down and reduced investment in daily living often lasts for a few weeks and ends gradually as a person begins to feel better. Schiff said that for her, as a bereaved parent, it meant cooking a meal. For another mother it was planting flowers, and for another actually applying for a job without "putting it off for another day."

Social Stresses

Many parents feel very much alone, particularly if they have lost an only child. Mothers often feel that there is no one who really understands. As one mother said, "How cruel can a person be? One woman had the nerve to tell me that I shouldn't be sad—after all, I had lost only one child, and I had two left." Such attempts to comfort may only make you feel more isolated, and it takes great courage to go back into regular social circles. Sometimes returning also means putting up with whispers behind your back and some awkward behavior from acquaintances.

The Problems of Making Changes at Home

As time passes some difficult decisions have to be made. Some parents find that they need several weeks or months before they can give away their children's belongings or make lasting alterations to their homes. Such delays are usually sensible. People who have just suffered a loss are vulnerable. Giving away treasures or making snap decisions such as selling a house are common mistakes that bereaved persons regret later on. In our experience we have found that those who have made such decisions usually have had the most difficulty facing their child's illness and accepting death. Perhaps their commonest need has been to renovate the dead child's room right after the funeral as if to banish painful memories instantly. On the other hand, a small number of parents have made a child's room into a shrine because they cannot get over the loss. This is equally sad.

Society's Difficulty with Death and How It Affects Parents

Today in our society we are faced with a number of difficulties that have accumulated because of our inability to face death. Public recognition of death, other than the tragedy of war, was banished between 1900 and 1970. For example, few children's books had any stories related to death, and the preferred location for death to occur moved from the home to the hospital around 1930. As we mentioned in Chapter 6, even cemeteries changed to parklike settings where death was hidden.

Unfortunately, such changes have meant that sorrow and grief have been seen as signs of mental instability, weakness, or bad manners, and fathers, in particular, have been expected to "keep a stiff upper lip." In addition, many young families have moved away from the extended family circle of grandparents, aunts, and uncles. These parents can no longer draw upon the valuable experiences of older adults when they have to face illness and death. By the same token, the failure of many young couples to continue religious practices has meant that this possible source of strength and comfort is no longer part of family life.

All of these factors mean that parents are inexperienced and alone when a child dies. Their ties to church are often weak, and people around them expect that they will "get their grief over quickly and get on with the job."

If relationships with your friends and relatives change, it may be helpful to remember how poorly prepared they are for death, especially the death of a child.

ABNORMAL GRIEF REACTIONS

Unfortunately, grief reactions can be distorted with some usually normal behaviors increasing in intensity and lasting for a long time. If you or your family see these changes in a family member or experience them yourselves, you may wish to make certain that the affected person obtains some much-needed counseling. Some of these distortions are described in the following sections.

Overactivity Without a Sense of Loss

After a death it is common to want to keep life going at home. Having things to do helps pass the time and makes mourning more tolerable. Friends and relatives often praise a mother who continues to be strong and keeps busy. Many times we have heard people admiring a bereaved mother: "She was so strong.", "What courage!", "Why, you'd never know her child just passed away." Unfortunately, such behavior usually leads to problems later on. For example, Mrs. M., the mother of Maria who had just died from leukemia, had been so busy she felt that she had to keep up the same pace after the funeral. She wrote all of her bereavement cards rapidly, cleaned the house from top to bottom, planted the garden, and never cried. After 2 or 3 weeks had passed she thought she was going to go insane. She had needed to remain strong for 2 years to help her child through the treatments. When her child died, in her words, "I could not let go and needed to keep moving." She no longer had her regular routine of driving many miles several times per week to bring her daughter for treatment, and she struggled to find a new routine at home. When she failed, her relationships with friends and family suffered and she felt that she couldn't think straight. Only after she sought professional help could she begin to let herself grieve.

Adopting the Symptoms of the Deceased

Occasionally when parents have a great deal of trouble adapting to their child's death, they are so anxious that they develop symptoms that their child experienced before death. Sometimes they even do this before death, and symptoms become worse afterwards. In one sad situation the mother of Angie, age 8, who died of a chest tumor, developed chest pains and palpitations (heavy heartbeats). She became increasingly preoccupied with her own health and pulled away from her friends and relatives.

She refused help from her doctor and withdrew from him as well. Between the first and second anniversaries of her child's death she became worse, and by the second anniversary she was hospitalized in a psychiatric unit, full of guilt and blaming herself for her child's death.

Psychosomatic Diseases

In some cases grief causes parents to develop new physical problems. Stress on their minds and bodies can occasionally result in such diseases as colitis (inflamed bowels), arthritis, and bronchial asthma. Although they happen only rarely, these diseases may be associated with anxiety, anger, and sadness.

How Intense Anger and Guilt Can Be Destructive

Although later sections on marital relationships and adjustment of siblings focus on relationship changes in detail, it is worth pointing out that anger and guilt play major roles in changing social and family relationships. When people are intensely angry and guilty differences are sharpened and major problems follow. Since guilt is hard to bear, it is easy to project it onto somebody else. For instance, one set of parents had fought for years but had stayed together for the benefit of their children. When their son, Angus, died at the age of 8, they blamed each other. Father's inability to handle the death was shown through his agitation and irrational behavior. He was under so much stress that he began to do strange things. At times he would vanish or race around the room or talk for hours without stopping. His wife directed so much of her own anger about their child's death toward him that he just could not handle it. For her, burdening her husband with the blame brought relief for herself.

It is common to feel cheated and angry when a child dies. Surprisingly, it is also common to feel angry with the child for dying. As the earlier example demonstrates, intense anger can be destructive. Many times parents want to be angry with God and have a very difficult time doing so. Part of their concern is that God will "get even." Thus, anger may be directed toward doctors or relatives because they are less threatening. Glenna, the 32-year-old mother of Jane, was a good example. Glenna was afraid of wide open spaces, of elevators, and of passing out. During psychiatric treatment she revealed that she worried that God would punish her if she was alone. He would do so because she was angry with Him and because she had allowed her daughter to become ill. Her turmoil reawakened anger from earlier days when she had been abandoned by her mother. Gradually, she began to direct this anger toward her mother at a time when her mother had difficulty understanding the reasons for her daughter's behavior. Without going further it is sufficient to say that Glenna's case was complex, but it serves to illustrate how anger can be destructive and how suffering can increase when old feelings are reawakened.

Sometimes anger can be misdirected for no apparent reason. One father, for example, just "blew up" at his boss. Minor irritations built up and he exploded in an outburst that almost cost him his job. Another father became involved in a fist fight when someone criticized him for making a minor mistake.

If people don't talk and express their feelings in acceptable ways such as playing sports, pounding nails, or talking, anger will creep out or burst forth in other ways. Turning anger inward can result in extreme guilt and problems like Glenna's or lead to a variety of relationship difficulties such as those just described.

Anxiety Can Be Overwhelming

Because of the uncertainty of cancer, parents are plagued with anxiety throughout their child's illness. Most manage to cope with it, and only a small number find it disabling. Sometimes people are naturally anxious anyway, and illness can heighten anxiety. After a child's death anxiety in small doses can be managed, and most parents who have been under continuous strain expect that it will take time to become calm and organized again. However, in a small number of cases anxiety will be overwhelming. Just as with anger, death may reawaken old anxieties and bring back feelings that have been forgotten since childhood. For example, part of Glenna's difficulty was her anxiety about what would happen to her and to her family. She was frightened of being by herself and of being hurt or mutilated. In some ways her fears were like the reawakening of feelings that she had when her mother had left her alone. She was vulnerable, helpless, and felt abandoned. When she worried constantly and was continually frightened she had trouble being the same helpful wife and mother that she had been before her child's illness and death. As she became more and more anxious she was afraid that she might die as well or that some other disaster would strike the family.

Depression: Problems Arise When Sadness Is Prolonged or Exaggerated

Another feeling that is common to grief is sadness. After a child's death nobody can blame a parent for being sad or tearful or even inactive for at least a week or two. Sometimes, however, sadness becomes more like a lasting depression, and certain symptoms or behavior patterns develop. For instance, loss of appetite, inability to go to sleep, or waking up early in the morning, slowness of speech and movement, speaking in monotones, disinterest in one's surroundings, excessive crying, and constantly having a long face and being unable to laugh or smile are all signs of depression. Taken alone, each of these symptoms can be expected to be part of any grief reaction. However, when they occur in combination and last for weeks on end it is wise to seek professional help.

For a small number of people who have a lasting depression and do not receive help, the consequences can be very serious. Depressed parents not only feel bad about themselves, but they also may begin to have fantasies that they too should die. They may want to rejoin their child, or they may feel that life is no longer worth living. Anniversaries of special events—particularly the anniversary of the child's death—are the most difficult and trying times for all bereaved parents. When a person is severely depressed such events can prove to be devastating.

Detrimental Acts: Hurt Can Make Some People Destroy Their Lives

Earlier we mentioned that people may do things that they regret later on. Sometimes, because of their upbringing and recent experience grieving parents are so upset that they want to destroy their lives or hurt themselves continually. Parents who turn to alcohol may use it to forget or to punish themselves or others. When they are drunk their personalities change, and they end up hurting those who are closest to them. Sometimes when parents cannot face what is happening they act impulsively, even without the influence of alcohol. A good example is selling the family home because it hurts too much to live there anymore. Sometimes people do "crazy things." One father bought up several businesses on credit all at once, only to regret his actions several days later.

It is important to recognize that when people do things that hurt themselves or their family they are usually in shock. If you or your partner or family see signs of this type of behavior, try to get the distressed person to your family physician or other source of help as quickly as possible. Many regrettable acts can be done in a hurry. Early recognition and assistance can save everyone the additional grief created by such mistakes.

If you can recognize the difference between "normal" and "abnormal" grief, your knowledge can be helpful when you try to understand your partner, your remaining children, and other relatives.

GRIEF AND MARRIAGES

You and Your Partner

Unfortunately, grieving is never easy. It is always associated with mental pain and suffering. People do not grieve in the same way or follow the same calendar. Parents who continue to share their lives together are faced with this problem each day. In most cases when a child is ill with cancer, grieving begins before the child dies, and if family problems occur during the last weeks or months of a child's life, they continue after death. Being sad, angry, or happy prior to death tends to be very much an individual matter. On days when a mother has felt sad a father may have felt angry, and so forth. After the child's death, because each person may grieve differently, couples frequently struggle to communicate and support each other emotionally. One mother told us that "When John thinks about the funeral he becomes sad and withdrawn, whereas I tend to reach out for him and cry. Because we are so different, we have actually helped each other—I draw him out and he comforts me." Another couple pointed out that when Margaret, age 7, was dying, they kept very busy. Father worked out his feelings through sports, and Mother would cry into her pillow. Their separate lives meant that Mother was most involved in Margaret's care. It was only after Margaret died that the couple came to realize that they had rarely shared their feelings together. It was hard for them because Father always hid his true feelings. It was only when he and his wife began to talk about their sadness that he began to realize that it was all right to cry in front of her. After this the couple drew closer, shared their sadness, and eventually began to reinvest themselves in continuing their lives together.

Sometimes parents are less fortunate and they begin to quarrel. It is easy to blame a partner for the death, especially if relatives side with one partner against the other. Inability to love and care for each other, failure to perform sexually, inability of one partner to work, pressure to pay medical bills, and a partner's abnormal grief reaction are other reasons why conflict develops. If marriage problems already exist grief can make them worse, and in extreme cases they force parents to separate. Unlike some other professionals, we do not believe that a child's death automatically causes marriage conflict and divorce. In fact, some couples find that they love and need each other even more because of what has happened to them and to their family.

Society's expectations of bereaved parents may add to the gulf between them. For instance, Father's work is an outlet for feelings, but it can become a permanent refuge and a way out of dealing with his grieving wife. On the other hand, work can be valuable therapy. The association with others, the tasks that provide a rest from memories, and the daily work routine can all help. They are most valuable when fathers combine the benefits of work with a need to share their feelings and talk openly about their loss, preferably with their partners.

As we discussed earlier it is difficult for a woman to reestablish herself at home and in the community. The process of mourning, complete with dreams, visions, and night noises, may mean that some mothers pine away the days. Being alone does not help, and husbands may not be willing or able to comfort or listen to them. When mothers have more time to think, sadness and anger increase and hurts deepen. For example, one mother said that every time she went out she became upset because "She just couldn't stand to see a normal child." It hurt her greatly, and it made her feel resentful that her only daughter had been "taken." When Father came home he found that she was so upset that he didn't know how to help her, so he just left her alone.

In another situation parents eventually shared their feelings, but only after Mother cried and suffered from headaches. Finally she found comfort by sitting in her child's room. She felt close to her there, and once Father got over his feelings of anger they recognized that they had been richer because their daughter had been so very much a part of their lives.

Should You Have More Children?

Along with the need to share feelings and to support each other comes the need to share in what may be lasting decisions. One common question is whether or not to have more children.

When a couple loses a child there is often a tendenc] want to fill the gap left by death. Many mothers who mo want to have another child. Most mothers recognize that they do not want a replica of their dead child but want another child who will receive the love that they have to give. For some, a new pregnancy is a way to prove themselves. They can show the world that they are capable of having healthy, normal children. For others it is a desire to start over, to fill the home with new life and reinvest themselves in motherhood. Others, at least at first, cannot bear facing the pain of worrying about whether or not they will experience another loss and are concerned that tragedy may hit twice. For a few these feelings are permanent, and they will never want to conceive again.

For young parents the advisability of new pregnancies or adopting depends upon the couple's recognition of why they want an additional child and at what point in their bereavement they are considering such an addition. We have found that it is wise for parents to wait at least 6 months or more and then discuss their needs with a professional whom they trust. For example, after 3-year-old Louise died of leukemia, Carol and Bob had one remaining daughter, age 6. After their second child was born, Bob had had a vasectomy. Shortly after Louise's death the couple were very lonely. They missed their daughter's company and her playful noises. Their other child, Cathy, went into Louise's room and cried. She held her sister's picture and was saddest at bedtime. Several friends, upon seeing their sadness, suggested that they should adopt another child. When they contacted a nurse from the pediatric cancer clinic, she suggested that they should wait a few months and then call the team's social worker. They did so several months later and at the time were certain that they wanted another child. With the social worker's help they explored the adoption possibilities, but he also pointed out that some vasectomies can be reversed. Gradually the couple decided to explore this possibility with their family doctor, and Bob proceeded to have the vasectomy reversed. Carol delivered a healthy baby boy 2 years later.

Setting New Priorities

Everyone likes to hear a happy story, and in fact Carol and Bob's experience does show how life can be reestablished. However, having more children is not the only way to reorganize family life. For some parents there is simply a need to reevaluate their priorities. One mother, Barbara, found that her whole life had changed. Housework took on a lower priority, and she found that she was now able to really "get to know Robbie all over again." Robbie, her 4-year-old son, had spent considerable time with neighbors and relatives, and Barbara felt that she had passed her responsibility on to them. As she put it, "I've begun to realize that Robbie is really a nice little boy—he's not such a brat after all." Atlhough Barbara said this with a great deal of humor, she felt that the pace of her life before her daughter's death had been so intense that her attention had to be focused on her sick child. After suffering the initial pains of loss, she began to spend much more time with Robbie and with her husband too.

Another mother, Andrea, was in tears after the death of her only son and came to see the clinic staff. She had been home for several months and could not bear the loneliness. She felt that only if she began work again could she really get over what had happened. The staff encouraged her and she started a new job. The association with co-workers helped her greatly, and at the end of a year she had moved through a normal pattern of grief.

UNDERSTANDING AND HELPING YOUR REMAINING CHILDREN

Listening

If you have read Chapter 6 you will recall that before age 8 or 9 children have considerable difficulty understanding the permanence of death. As a parent of young children you need to recognize that in order for them to understand what has happened they must be allowed to talk about death and ask questions. Sometimes such discussion can be very painful for you, but it is a necessary step for them. Problems for brothers and sisters occur most frequently when parents close the door on discussion. This is dealt with in detail later on in this section.

How Children Differ from Adults

When young children mourn they move in and out of sadness quickly. It is not unusual for them to be tearful one moment and to laugh and play in the next. It is also common for them to ask one or two questions, listen for the answer, and run off to play again. This behavior can be upsetting to adults, particularly older adults. Adult thinking dictates that a person should be sad, tearful, and serious. The hushed voices at the funeral home, dressing in black, and sitting at a wake have become less customary, but the fact remains that many older persons expect people to suffer from the loss. This expectation just doesn't fit young children, at least not for more than a minute or two at a time. They are lively, active, and playful and must try to fit sadness and loss into the pattern of their behavior. They usually lack the experience of previous losses and are not able to fit the concept of time into most of their experiences.

For some parents young children are a blessing, because they are demanding and full of bounce and they relieve the sadness of the adult world. As one mother said, "Without the other two young ones, I never would have made it. I had to go on living for them, and their constant activity really helped me."

Play Can Help Children Grieve

Relief through play and the chance to work out their feelings in their own way help children to return to Mom and Dad or Grandma or Grandpa to clarify other questions. They want short, understandable answers. As Schiff pointed out in her book, she had to help her 4-year-old understand why her brother had died. She finally told her that he was no longer in pain. This explanation was one that her daughter could understand.

Young children, even when they have the chance to speak openly of death, still find it to be very difficult. For instance, for a couple of weeks after his sister's death Jason, age 4, was playing and acting normally. One day he broke out in a rash and began to scream. After his outburst his parents learned that he had suddenly realized that his sister was not coming back to sleep in her room. He missed her desperately and the permanence of her death hit home, at least temporarily. The comfort of his parents helped. Later on they noticed that he and his cousin were planting a make-believe garden and incorporating his sister into their play. She was planting her garden in Heaven and doing the same things that they were.

Fantasy and Magic

Children's greatest advantage in managing grief is their ability to use fantasy. The imaginary world relieves some of the pain and suffering of the real world and makes threatening things

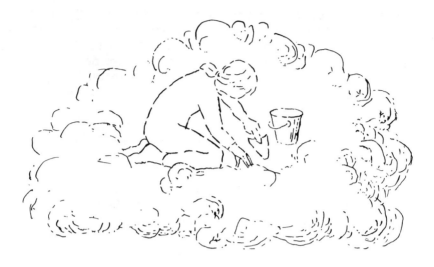

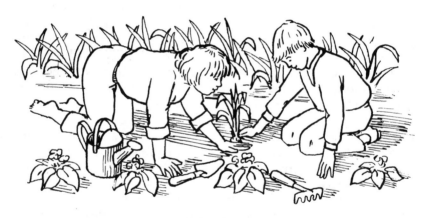

harmless. If you recall from Chapter 6, one little boy imagined he could hook a ladder to the clouds and go to see his sister in Heaven. Another decided that his sister was an angel and believed that she watched over him. At night he would talk to her.

Children, in their world of imagination and magic, believe that dead people can hear. Consequently they want to talk with them, both at times of play and on visits to the cemetery. If you stop to think about it, some of these beliefs and behaviors continue into adult life. Many adults go to a cemetery and talk to the grave and find it comforting.

Sometimes when children have religious beliefs they find comfort in the idea that a dead person is being cared for. For some it may be that Grandma or Grandpa is in Heaven with their brother or sister. Others may believe that God or Jesus is providing care or comfort. Many children want to be reassured that after death more exists than just being buried and being left in the ground to decay.

It is worth remembering that many needs and behaviors of young children carry over to later life, and fantasy can creep back into beliefs of older children and adolescents as well. Even the realistic thought pattern of a 10- or 12-year-old may be skewed by fantasy at times of stress. Although it is most common for young children to feel guilty about having caused or contributed to death, it can also be a problem for older children.

Grief and Older Children

When older children see a brother or sister die they often worry that they may die as well. Older children grieve in a similar manner to adults and feel the loss intensely. They hurt and feel guilty. "If I had only . . ." If their parents are anxious, older children may wonder whether or not they can contract the same disease. Some worry that they may die when they reach the same age as their older brother or sister was at the time of his or her death. Again, these feelings are not just confined to older children but carry over into adolescence as well.

The Adolescent

For adolescents, the death of a sibling occurs at a time when they are trying to establish their identity. Who are they? What will they become? Will they grow up at all? Adolescents tend to be self-centered, and their need to establish themselves leads them into conflict with their parents on their path to independence. Brooding, loneliness, and anxiety are natural, and the death of a brother or sister increases the intensity of such feelings. Sometimes adolescents become remote and uncommunicative. They retreat in order to sort out what death means. The death of a brother or sister can lead to outbursts of anger when emotions well up and burst forth. Sometimes such anger seems entirely unrelated to the death, stems from a trivial matter, and is directed at someone who had absolutely nothing to

,h the loss. Sometimes, in order to protect themselves, 1g adolescents will use denial much in the same way as nd dying adolescents do. Denying what has happened and reinvesting in life, sometimes at a very hectic pace, is a way of forgetting that is much less painful than dwelling on memories.

In mourning, as in normal living, natural gaps between parent and adolescent must exist. As we suggested earlier, the rituals surrounding death are frequently rejected by adolescents. The fact that Mother may continuously mourn for several weeks or months is also distressing because she constantly reminds the adolescent of the pain of the loss. Sometimes this is just too much to handle, and some adolescents escape or rebel.

Other Problems for Siblings

Everyone in the family grieves. Age matters little. Irritability, prolonged tearfulness, or withdrawal are common. So also is the development of minor physical problems—stomach aches and headaches are those seen most frequently. Difficulties in school are also common. For most siblings a decline in school performance for a few months is to be expected. Bouts of daydreaming are normal. These are characterized by preoccupation with what has happened and speculation about what will become of the family. If, however, the decline is lasting and children become disinterested and listless in school, they are probably depressed and professional help is in order.

If parents have difficulty coping and life at home remains unsettled, some children may not begin to grieve for several months or even years. As an example, Les was the ideal little boy when his sister died. One year later he suddenly became disruptive in school and refused to do his work. His unexpected change in behavior was puzzling to his parents and teachers. Such delayed reactions may be avoided if parents can manage their own grief and reestablish family life soon after a child's death. This will allow the remaining children to work through their own grief.

Keeping Communication Lines Open

As parents you have a difficult task sorting out what is reasonable to expect and what is "abnormal." It is easy to say that parents should communicate with their children about what has happened, but it may not be easy to do so. This is especially true when children don't wish to talk.

Since mourning is a very personal experience, it may be quite reasonable for you to give your children time to sort their feelings out for themselves. Sometimes they do such sorting well by using brothers and sisters or friends. Perhaps the most important factor for you to recognize is that you should not banish the subject of their dead brother or sister from daily life. It is not wise to dwell on the loss, but the gap that your dead child has left cannot and should not go unnoticed.

If a children's bereavement support group is available in your area, your children may benefit by sharing their feelings and working through their loss.*

THE FAMILY

How Families React

Since the pace of mourning varies for everyone in the family, life can become complicated. Mrs. S., the single parent of Al, who died a year ago, said her biggest problem was that she had to work through her own feelings of loss before she could help her other two children. This took several months, and by that time Dick, age 7, wouldn't talk about his brother's death. Dick was irritable and lashing out at other children in the neighborhood. In another family, Mrs. J. found that she had little chance to work out her own feelings and communicate with her husband because her own brothers and sisters kept bringing their problems to her. They had severe difficulties arising from their inability to accept their nephew's death and felt that they could inflict their concerns on her just as they had always done in the past.

Some very specific problems can arise between parents and remaining children. Each child has played an important part in family life. Everyone in the family fulfills certain purposes and carries out specific tasks. Individuals may perform several roles. For instance, being thoughtful, caring, or humorous may be characteristic of one or several members. Others may offer discipline, provide foresight, or be the organizers or philosophers in the family.

When children die it is very common for parents to want to remember all of their children's best qualities. They magnify the good qualities to make their children into ideal persons. In some ways this thinking serves to unconsciously justify the deepness of their loss and the disruption in their lives. In small doses such behavior is reasonable. If, however, such idolization goes unchecked and continues to increase, major problems arise for other children.

* see Appendix E: Siblings' Bereavement Groups p. 297.

Idolizing and Replacing a Child

It is fair to say that no child is replaceable. Each child is unique, and the love that parents have provided has been for him or her as an individual. Idolizing, however, frequently means that the remaining children are faced with the problem of never quite living up to the standards set by dead children. Some parents may wish to deny it, but the fact remains that most compare the qualities and performance of all of their children. Ways to compare arise naturally—school performance and ability at sports are common examples. When parents are grieving they have to be careful that their mourning does not lead them to try to artificially fill the gap left by a deceased child. For example, ability to play baseball may never be the strength of a remaining child, and Father must recognize it. In other words, you cannot make over your remaining children to fulfill your needs and heal your wounds.

Overprotecting Remaining Children

When parents lose one child the remaining child or children become especially valuable. Parents who lose a child often become much more protective of their other children. The increase in rules and discipline that can result may be resented by children who remain, especially if these are tied to the death of their brother or sister. Sometimes such changes increase their anger toward the dead child for leaving and making life unbearable. After all, life has changed for the worst, and now their freedoms and pleasures are being severely reduced. Overprotecting shows up in other ways too. Frequently, bereaved mothers will watch over their healthy children and bring them to cancer treatment centers. They bypass the family doctor because they are so worried that cancer might strike twice. Constant checking of remaining children can make them very anxious and upset. In a small number of cases these children may develop their own imaginary symptoms. Even when parents are just slightly protective, the fear that they might get cancer and die is very prominent in surviving siblings.

Keeping Silent

Several times we have mentioned the need to allow the subject of a deceased child's contribution to the family to remain part of family life. This is to avoid the "haunting" that can occur if remaining children are not allowed to talk over their feelings about their loss. Several times we have seen teenagers and young adults who have been very upset because a discussion or event has brought back memories of the death of a sibling. One medical student, discussing a case, suddenly began to cry. A film he had just seen reminded him of the death of his sister 10 years before. Whenever he had tried to talk about it his parents had changed the subject. He felt responsible and angry. He did not know exactly what had happened and felt that he was being deserted. These feelings were filed in the back of his mind and apparently forgotten. Gradually, as he began to express them, he recognized what had happened to him and he began to feel better. In another situation, a mother told us about her 15-year-old's "nervous breakdown." He became agitated, depressed, and intensely angry at his father. Finally he let everyone in the family know that he was upset because, 9 years before, his parents had completely wiped his brother's existence out of their lives without a trace. After the death his brother's grave was not visited, his room was quickly remodeled, his toys disappeared, and his father would not allow the dead child's name to be mentioned again. In addition, his father developed an ulcer and became ill-tempered. For 9 years the boy had felt rejected, and finally he could no longer bear the silence.

New Children

In closing this section it is important to note that family members will fill the gaps left by the deceased child. This occurs naturally, and often changes come slowly and subtly. It is the extremes in behavior that create the problems, and awareness of these should be helpful. We have not, however, dealt with the birth of a new child. This subject is worth mentioning, at least briefly.

For some parents pregnancy while a child is dying, or shortly after, may seem sensible. Mothers become preoccupied with a new life, and the pain of loss may be reduced. It seems that having this new infant to love should make life easier. In reality this may not be the case. If a child is dying the stress of a new pregnancy and the anxiety it generates may add to fear already existing about illness and death. If a child has died the pregnancy may interrupt or impede the mourning process. For instance, it has been demonstrated that mothers who lose a baby and become pregnant again in the 6 months following have a more difficult time with grief reactions.

In rare instances parents who have severe difficulties with grief reactions may create problems for their new child. One sad example occurred when 10-year-old Joanna died. Several months later when the mother became pregnant she gave her new baby daughter the same name. The parents idolized the new baby and treated her as if she were the same child as the Joanna who died. Studies have shown that children who have been "cast in the same image"* as their deceased sibling have developed severe psychological problems.

The Strength of the Family and Help from Professionals

In each family time will help heal the wounds of grief. If you are faced with a child's death you may find that the natural love, affection, and caring that is already present in your family may help the most. Learning to use and build on your own strengths and those of other family members can result in great accomplishments. You may find that with the support of friends, neighbors, clergy, family doctors, and others your family will move through the mourning period successfully. This is especially true if you have faced some of your grief before your child died. However, if you need help, do not hesitate to seek it. It is better to ask for assistance early on than to be plagued with trying to sort out severe emotional difficulties later. In some cities groups such as the Candlelighters or other organizations for bereaved parents such as The Compassionate Friends, Inc. offer comfort through association with other parents who have been through the same experience. Often the feeling that you are not alone helps greatly, or sometimes it is simply knowing what is ahead that will help you face the future. If your problems are severe, however, family doctors may help by referring you to psychiatric resources. Reestablishment of contact with the nurse or social worker at the cancer treatment center may also be helpful.

Help from Friends, Neighbors, and the Hospital

Earlier, when discussing the time of the funeral, we mentioned the fact that friends and relatives often do not know how to

*A. C. Cain & B. S. Cain, "On Replacing a Child." *American Journal of the Academy of Child Psychiatry,* 1964, 3, 444.

react. Most parents, however, have found that there are one or two or even more persons who prove to be invaluable. They are helpful because they remain close but allow parents to be themselves. As one couple put it, "Our real friends were two couples whom we could phone up and ask to come over to the house. They would always come, and we could say 'Tell us if you think we are going crazy,' or 'Please don't talk about our problems tonight, let's just play cards.' These friends were the ones who helped us take care of our other children, who went with us to the funeral home, and helped us to keep our home going when we just couldn't mow the lawn or water the flowers." In other situations this type of support has been offered by grandparents or other relatives. One couple used Grandma as a gauge to tell them how the family was managing. She had always been warm and caring, and the couple trusted her for her fairness and wisdom. She helped them through every part of their grief reaction.

In certain situations such help has come from outsiders—Cancer Society volunteers, family doctor, hospital staff, the clergy, or the congregation from a church. Many times parents have returned to the hospital to obtain autopsy results or to see specific staff. At our center we always set aside time for such visits, and on many occasions parents have told us how much they have felt as if we were part of their family and, in turn, they were part of the hospital family. We believe that most people in hospitals care and that if time allows such brief encounters are helpful. Staff like to feel that families are "doing all right" and enjoy the renewal of what was often a close relationship. We believe that families do not need to grieve alone. Help is available; if you need it, seek it out. If assistance is required, hospital staff can usually provide it.

When Relatives Are a Burden

Like Mrs. S., Al's mother, some parents are plagued by emotionally needy relatives or friends. This creates a terrible dilemma. As a parent you are hurt, and you know what it is like. You know it is hard for others in the family, and you know the past history of what has happened to them. For example, they may have "fallen apart" when your mother died or taken to drinking heavily. Perhaps because you are a strong person, others have always relied on you to comfort and care for them. Sons and daughters feel this way sometimes when parents are aged and suffering.

The problem is that right now you just don't need the stress of their demands. In fact, you may not be able to manage their problems and still carry on with your own grieving. What do you do? Do you become the cruel relative—the one who has lost a child and has no feelings left for the rest of the family?

In this situation no one can tell you what to do. Most of the time, though, when bereaved parents are firm and tell these needy persons the truth, they are successful in directing them elsewhere for help. The point is that you usually have to sort out your own feelings before you can help others, so, for the time being at least, someone else can probably be more helpful to them.

Coping with Anniversaries

Birthdays, the date of a child's death, the date of diagnosis, Christmas, Easter, and other special days during the year can all bring back memories and renew old hurts. These days may be filled with feelings of loss and sadness and may be a time to feel depressed. On the other hand, they may also be times that are filled with pleasant memories of all of the happy events you experienced with your child while he or she was living. Unfortunately it is necessary for you to experience both the positive and negative feelings as part of grieving. If you are dreading an anniversary it is usually helpful to be with other people. They care as well and can offer you comfort, consolation, and diversion at a time when you need it most.

Unfortunately some parents have reported that some companies and organizations have tried to prey upon their sadness at a time close to the first anniversary of their child's death. These commercial enterprises try to encourage parents to "enshrine" their child by spending money on elaborate plaques or other reminders. Most parents have found the practice revolting.

SOME THOUGHTS FOR SINGLE PARENTS

Needs Immediately Following Death

In our experience the most important need for single parents is to have someone to talk to about their feelings and to review with them the importance of their child's life. This discussion of feelings is usually best done with friends, with other parents whose children have died, or with professionals who understand bereavement. This is mainly because other family members often have unreasonable expectations about the nature and length of grief reactions and because these family members are grieving themselves. When they grieve they may do so in a very different way from a single parent, and because of their sorrow they may be poor listeners. If you are in this position you may find that you are so upset that you wonder if you are going "crazy." Contact with outsiders can be helpful because their reassurance that you are not mentally ill will probably mean more than if it comes from family members. Other bereaved parents and professionals can also be reassuring because they help you learn that others have suffered in the same way. Such contact also removes the overwhelming feelings of loneliness that usually follow before single parents can reestablish themselves.

Caring for Your Other Children

When you are alone not only do you lack a partner to confide in but you also lack a person with whom to share the responsibility of helping your other children work through their feelings of loss. This can mean that you may unwillingly neglect your other children because you are so wrapped up in your own problems and overwhelmed by your feelings. As one single parent described it, "My youngest son, Dwayne, was all right for a while after Jake's death. A few months later he began having problems in school and became extremely irritable. He would blow up at the drop of a hat. I only realized recently that I had to try so hard to cope with my own feelings of loss that I hadn't been able to help him." She continued by explaining that she had now begun to reinvest herself by upgrading her education in preparation for work and was now able to help her son.

Fortunately Dwayne's mother recognized that he also was grieving and was prepared to assist him even if her assistance was delayed. Other parents may be less observant and blame such unexpected behavior on other causes. Children suffer from having only one parent to confide in. In single-parent families if they are unable to discuss their feelings with a remaining parent they may keep their emotions and thoughts bottled up inside. They do so because they know that their mother or father is upset and they don't want to make the situation worse. As a result some single parents have found that selected friends, relatives, and grandparents may be helpful if they are close to the remaining children and can talk about death openly. In our experience, when problems have been severe family physicians and hospital staff from child life, social work, and nursing have been helpful. Much depends on whether or not children feel that they can trust a specific adult and whether or not the adult can communicate with children in ways that they accept and understand.

Sometimes the relationship with other adults is most helpful when they are of the opposite sex to that of the single parent. For instance, young boys may find it easier to speak with their grandfather than with their mother. As children pass through various stages of development there are times that they relate more easily to members of the opposite sex and times when they are more attached to a member of the same sex.

Anniversaries

We mentioned earlier that anniversaries of a child's death or birthday are upsetting for almost all parents. Single parents are no exception. In fact they usually need other people to provide companionship and emotional support even more than in families where both parents are present. Some have worried that they will have a "nervous breakdown" because they are frightened of reliving the child's death in their memories. Fortunately most manage well. It may be worthwhile for you to recognize that such anniversaries are upsetting so that you can plan to be with friends or relatives.

FOR EVERY PARENT

In closing this chapter it is important to remember that most parents do survive their child's death and remain healthy themselves. Although the year or so of grieving following your child's death is a time of suffering, it should lead to healing and renewal. As you continue to remember your child, most likely the pain of cancer and death will dull and you will remember the blessings of life that were so much a part of the years when your child was alive.

Many parents have said that they have gained from their suffering despite the pain and anguish. They have found that they have learned to appreciate themselves and the qualities of

their friends and family. Many have found solace in the belief
that their child was loaned to them by God, and gradually time
has healed over the wounds of illness and death.

Claire Mulholland says it well in this poem:

> I am not glad you suffered
> That would be mockery
> But I can accept now
> That it has happened
> And be glad.
>
> Because of you
> I am part of the World's hurts
> And am at one with each.
>
> Because of you
> Each moment is precious
> And nothing is taken for granted.
>
> Because of you
> I have found joy and depth
> And Laughter
>
> Because you died
> My beautiful daughter.

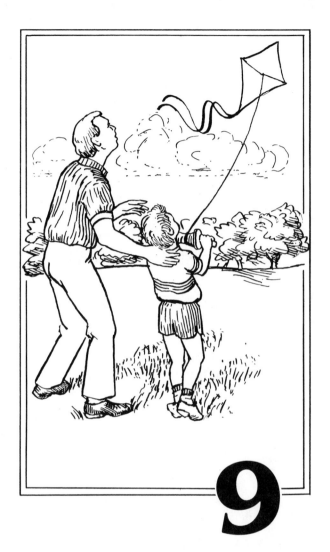

9

NEW IDEAS,
NEW DIRECTIONS

As we have attempted to guide you through the problems of coping with childhood cancer, we have kept our focus as practical as possible. However, we could not close out our work without bringing to your attention some recent approaches to thinking about cancer and attempting to overcome it.

HOLISTIC APPROACH TO CANCER TREATMENT

In recent years the literature regarding cancer and cancer treatment has contained increased reference to a linkage between the mind and body. In fact, a school of belief in a holistic approach to illness and well-being has developed. The underlying idea is that, for adults at least, serious illnesses such as cancer are related to the whole person. The mind, spirit, emotions, and lifestyle of those afflicted are all factors that are believed to contribute to the development and recurrence of cancer as well as the recovery from it. Some of those who believe in holistic treatment propose that those who have cancer must change their approach to life, and particularly their mental attitude. The development of a positive and relaxed outlook coupled with a determination to conquer this disease is said to replace overwhelming feelings of despair and hopelessness. In practice, some holistic treatment programs include a great deal of emotional support and a specific pattern of changing one's outlook in order to help the body promote healing. These programs are often given in combination with traditional medical treatment.

There is more than one approach in holistic medicine. One technique uses imagery, that is, picturing the cancer within the body in an attempt to control or overcome it. It has not been proven that this technique will increase a person's chances of survival. However, some adult patients have said that they have felt more hopeful and more in control of what is happening to their bodies.

Other techniques of holistic treatment operate on the philosophy that love is the most important healing force. Attitudinal healing focuses on the choice of peace as opposed to conflict and love rather than fear. The principles involved include the recognition that health is "letting go of fear" and finding "inner peace." It is believed that people can give to others, be happy inside, and view other persons as givers of love or seekers of help. *

THE VALUE OF THE APPROACH

There is a growing collection of examples of persons who have managed their illness better or lived beyond current expectations because they have changed their attitude and lifestyle. When such changes are in harmony with existing medical treatment cancer patients may gain in their ability to endure the side effects of treatment, fight off their disease, and go on living. There is no doubt that teaching people to relax and gain self control is worthwhile.

At present the holistic approach is not apt to be found in every community, and in fact it will not appeal to everyone. The efficacy of the techniques of holistic medicine is far from being proven. Nevertheless, there is an underlying relationship between the idea of the holistic approach and what is offered in this book. We believe that knowledge helps to reduce fear. We also believe that the positive attitudes of parents and their ability to help their children are extremely important in completing treatment and helping recovery. When children are relaxed and happy quality is maintained in their lives. We think that the new ideas for helping to overcome illness should continue to be tested and evaluated. We do not have any specific beliefs on how much stress contributes to childhood cancer. We think that considerable research is required before such a linkage can be proved. For the present, we know that stress for the child must be controlled as much as possible and that for those in relapse it seems that maintaining the will to live is very important.

* Deliman, T., & Smolowe, J. S. *Holistic Medicine: Harmony of Body, Mind, Spirit.* Reston VA: Reston Publishing Company, 1982, pp. 87, 192, 214, 228, 260.

IN CLOSING

As we conclude this book it is our hope that you will be encouraged to draw your family together, to increase the amount of communication between you and your family, and to find the strength to cope with the crises of cancer and go on living.

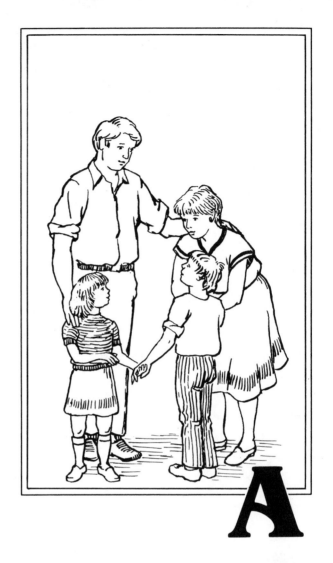

A
CHEMOTHERAPY AND
ITS SIDE EFFECTS

Chemotherapy is the use of anticancer drugs to destroy malignant cells within your child's body. A variety of drugs may be used during the course of your child's treatment. They may be given in several different forms. Some drugs may be taken daily as pills. Others may be given intravenously (IV), intramuscularly (IM), or subcutaneously (SC). Certain drugs may be given intrathecally (into the spinal canal) to treat brain tumors or to prevent or treat central nervous system leukemia.

Pills are usually given at home. This can sometimes be a problem for younger children. Most of these medications can be broken into smaller pieces or crushed into a powder and mixed with honey, jam, or applesauce for easier swallowing. If your child experiences any difficulties taking his or her medication discuss it with your child's physician.

It is important for parents to be familiar with the medications their children are taking. It is also helpful for you and your child to keep track of these medications. Some parents find it useful to keep a record on a calendar and bring it with them to regular clinic visits.

The most common anticancer drugs, their description, action, route, and side effects are listed in the drug chart at the end of this appendix.

SIDE EFFECTS OF CHEMOTHERAPY

All anticancer drugs are designed to kill malignant cells. Some drugs interfere with cell division while others interfere with the chemical processes inside of the cells. Eventually the cancer cells are destroyed.

These drugs also affect normal cells to some extent. Cells that divide rapidly such as those in the bone marrow, hair follicles, and the gastrointestinal tract, are disturbed and some are destroyed. As a result there are often side effects. These can be upsetting but are usually temporary and reversible.

Important Points About Side Effects

1. One of the most common side effects of chemotherapy is *bone marrow depression*. This means the bone marrow's ability to produce adequate numbers of blood cells is reduced. If red cells are low there is a possibility of anemia. A decrease of platelets increases the possibility of bleeding. A low white cell count may put your child at a greater risk for infection. Therefore, it is important to watch for signs of bruising, bleeding, or infection.

2. *Most side effects are reversible.* Some may improve as chemotherapy continues. Stopping the drug for a time may improve other side effects.

3. *Side effects vary from child to child and even from treatment to treatment.* Your child may experience some or none of the side effects associated with any particular drug. Parents have found it important to be aware of the reactions that may occur so that they have a better understanding of what to expect and can recognize any symptoms quickly.

4. *Persistent, unacceptable side effects may be altered by decreasing the dosage of the drug.* This does not usually reduce the drug's ability to control the cancer. Parents should not be alarmed because the dose has changed.

5. Certain drugs such as Actinomycin D, Adriamycin, BCNU, and Cyclophosphamide may *increase the effects of radiation*. This is usually beneficial; however, it may also produce more side effects.

6. Some reactions may occur immediately (acute) while others may develop days or weeks after the medication has been given (delayed). Nausea and vomiting are common acute side effects. Hair loss and bone marrow depression are common delayed side effects.

Ways to Control or Prevent Certain Side Effects

1. *Nausea and vomiting* are caused by many anticancer drugs. Medication that is available may help to reduce the severity of this reaction but may not totally prevent it. It has been

found that medication is most beneficial when given before chemotherapy. Some treatment centers use relaxation exercises and hypnosis to help counteract these symptoms.

2. *Sore mouth and mouth ulcers* can be eased by a special mouthwash prescribed by your child's physician. It should be used regularly, and your child should rinse his or her mouth well after each meal. Q-tips™, glycerin swabs, or a very soft toothbrush should be used to remove food particles. Painful mouth sores may be relieved by applying a local anesthetic prescribed by your child's doctor. This may make it easier for your child to eat, and it should be applied just before meal time.

3. *Heartburn or stomachaches* from Prednisone or Dexamethasone can usually be prevented by giving one-half glass of milk with each dose of drug.

4. *Weight gain and elevated blood pressure* from Prednisone or Dexamethasone can be controlled to some extent by avoiding very fatty foods and limiting the addition of salt to food. It is also helpful to avoid salty snacks such as potato chips, pretzels, and so on.

5. *Tissue burns* can occur when Vincristine, Adriamycin, and other drugs have leaked at the site of injection. If this happens at the time of injection cold compresses are applied. If redness, swelling, and pain develop within a few days after injection your child's doctor should be notified. Prompt treatment may prevent a severe burn or ulceration of the skin.

6. *Hair loss* can occur from Adriamycin, Cyclophosphamide, Methotrexate, and Vincristine. There is no simple effective way to prevent this from occurring except to discontinue the medication. Because of the beneficial effects of these drugs, hair loss is considered to be an acceptable side effect. For further discussion please refer to the section on hair loss in Chapter 3.

7. *Hemorrhagic cystitis* can develop from Cyclophosphamide. This is irritation and bleeding in the bladder. To decrease the possibility of this problem developing, the drug should be prevented from remaining in the bladder for a long time. Your child should receive the drug early in the day and then, to increase urination, he or she must be encouraged to drink more fluids throughout the day. The amount of liquids the child takes depends on his or her size, so this should be discussed with your doctor. Do *not* rely on your child's thirst

to determine intake. If you notice pink or bloody urine any time after treatment you should contact your child's physician as soon as possible. In most centers an additional amount of fluid is administered before your child is sent home.

When You Should Call the Doctor

You should notify your child's doctor when you see:

1. Allergic reactions such as hives, swelling of hands, feet, and eyelids.

2. Excessive bruising or bleeding. Remember that signs of bleeding may also be seen in urine (pink, red, brownish) and in stools (red or black).

3. Shortness of breath while taking Daunomycin, Adriamycin, or Methotrexate.

4. Excessive thirst or urination while taking Prednisone or Dexamethasone.

5. Extreme weakness after completing Prednisone or Dexamethasone.

6. Blood in urine and pain during or after taking Cyclophosphamide.

7. Jaundice (a yellow tinge to the skin and eyeballs) while taking any medication.

8. Exposure to a contagious disease, especially chicken pox or measles, unless you know your child is immune to these.

9. Fever or any sign of infection that persists or becomes worse.

10. Persistent headaches.

11. Reddened or swollen areas.

12. Any problems with eyesight such as blurred or double vision.

13. Unexpected vomiting, especially if it is not associated with radiation or chemotherapy.

Please recognize that this list relates to major concerns. Your child's physician may advise you of others. If you are in doubt you should feel free to ask for advice.

SOME COMMON MEDICATIONS USED IN TREATING CHILDHOOD CANCER

Medication	Description	Action	Route Given	Frequency	Possible Side Effects	Incidence	Precautions
Actinomycin-D (Dactinomycin, Cosmegen)	Clear yellow liquid	Antibiotic that inhibits formation of DNA and RNA.	IV	Variable	Nausea, vomiting Bone marrow depression Hair loss Skin eruptions (acne) Fever	F F O R R	May cause tissue burns if it infiltrates. May increase side effects of radiation.
Adriamycin (Doxorubicin)	Clear red liquid	Antibiotic that inhibits formation of DNA and RNA.	IV	Variable	Nausea, vomiting Hair loss Pink urine (not blood) Bone marrow depression Mouth ulcers Fever Heart damage	F F F F F O R	Causes tissue burns if it infiltrates. Echocardiogram should be done at regular intervals.
Allopurinol (Zyloprim)	Tablet White:100 mg Peach:300 mg	Prevents formation of uric acid (waste product of leukemic cells).	Oral	Daily	Nausea, vomiting Diarrhea Rash	O O R	

NOTE: For more specific information about the dosage, action, side effects, and methods of administration you should consult your child's physician.

KEY: IV—Intravenously; IM—Intramuscularly; IT—intrathecally (into spinal canal); SC—subcutaneously (under skin); F—frequent; O—occasional; R—rare.

Medication	Description	Action	Route Given	Frequency	Possible Side Effects	Incidence	Precautions
BCNU (Carmustine)	Clear colorless liquid	Reacts with and damages nucleus of rapidly growing cells.	IV	Usually 6–8 week intervals	Nausea, vomiting (1–6 hours after injection)	F	Pulmonary (lung) function tests should be done regularly.
					Bone marrow depression (3–4 weeks after injection)	F	
					Mild liver injury	O	
					Burning along vein during injection	O	
Bleomycin (Blenoxane)	Clear colorless liquid	Inhibits formation of DNA.	IV IM SC	Variable	Nausea, vomiting	F	Pulmonary (lung) function tests should be done regularly.
					Fever, chills at time of injection	F	
					Mouth ulcers	F	
					Hair Loss	F	
					Loss of appetite and weight	F	
					Allergic reaction (3–5 hours after injection)	R	
					Liver and kidney damage	R	
Busulfan (Myleran)	Small white scored tablet: 2 mg	Reacts with and damages nucleus of rapidly growing marrow cells.	Oral	Daily	Bone marrow depression	F	
					Nausea, vomiting	O	
					Diarrhea	O	
					Sore mouth	O	
					Increased skin pigmentation	R	

Drug	Form	Action	Route	Schedule	Side Effects		Administration
CCNU (Lomustine)	Capsules: 10, 40, 100 mg	Reacts with and damages nucleus of rapidly growing cells.	Oral	Usually 6-8 week intervals	Nausea, vomiting	F	Give with small amount of water on empty stomach then nothing to eat or drink for 2 hours.
					Bone marrow depression (3-6 weeks after dose)	F	
					Mild liver injury	O	
Chlorambucil (Leukeran)	White sugar-coated tablet: 2 mg.	Inhibits formation of DNA and RNA.	Oral	Variable	Nausea, vomiting	F	
					Loss of appetite	F	
					Bone marrow depression	F	
Cis-Platinum	Clear colorless liquid	Toxic to rapidly growing cells.	IV	Variable	Nausea, vomiting may be severe	F	
					Loss of appetite	F	
					Bone marrow depression	F	
					Kidney damage	R	
Cyclophosphamide (Cytoxan Procytox)	Colorless liquid White pill with blue flecks Medium: 25 mg Large: 50 mg	Reacts with and damages nucleus of rapidly growing cells.	IV Oral	Variable	Nausea, vomiting	F	Give large amount of fluids to prevent cystitis.
					Loss of appetite	F	
					Hair loss	F	
					Bone marrow depression	F	
					Mouth ulcers	O	
					Cystitis (bladder inflammation with blood in urine)	O	
					Diarrhea	R	
					Liver injury	R	

NOTE: For more specific information about the dosage, action, side effects, and methods of administration you should consult your child's physician.

Medication	Description	Action	Route Given	Frequency	Possible Side Effects	Incidence	Precautions
Cytosine Arabinoside (Ara-C, Cytarabine, Cytosar)	Clear colorless liquid	Inhibits DNA production.	IV SC IT	Variable	Nausea, vomiting	F	
					Loss of appetite	F	
					Bone marrow depression	F	
					Abdominal cramps	O	
					Diarrhea	O	
					Sore mouth and throat	O	
					Headache	R	
					Liver damage	R	
Daunomycin (Daunorubicin, Rubidomycin)	Clear red liquid	Antibiotic that inhibits formation of DNA and RNA.	IV	Variable	Nausea, vomiting	F	Causes tissue burns if it infiltrates.
					Bone marrow depression	F	
					Pink urine (not blood)	F	
					Hair loss	F	
					Mouth ulcers	O	
					Fever	O	Echocardiogram should be done at regular intervals.
					Heart damage	R	
Dexamethasone (Decadron)	Small, 5-sided colored pill	See Prednisone.					
Dacarbazine (DTIC)	Clear yellowish liquid	Toxic to rapidly dividing cells.	IV	Variable	Bone marrow depression	F	
					Burning along vein of injection	F	
					Nausea, vomiting	O	
					Fever	O	

Drug	Form	Action	Route	Schedule	Side effects	Notes
Hydroxyurea (Hydrea)	Capsule: 500 mg (green & pink)	Inhibits production of DNA.	Oral	Variable	Bone marrow depression (F), Nausea, vomiting (O), Mouth ulcers (O), Headache, dizziness (R), Skin rash (R), Mouth ulcers (R)	May increase side effects of radiation.
L-Asparaginase (Elspar, Kidrolase)	Thick colorless liquid	Starves leukemic cells and prevents them from manufacturing protein.	IM IV SC	Variable	Loss of appetite (F), Tiredness (F), Nausea, vomiting (O), Fever (O), Allergic reactions may be severe (O), Liver or pancreas dysfunction (abdominal pain, high blood sugar, increased thirst and urination) (R)	
6-Mercaptopurine (6MP, Purinethol)	Large white tablet: 50 mg	Inhibits production of proteins.	Oral	Daily	Bone marrow depression (F), Nausea, vomiting (O), Loss of appetite (O), Diarrhea (R), Fever (R), Mouth ulcers (R)	

NOTE: For more specific information about the dosage, action, side effects, and methods of administration you should consult your child's physician.

Medication	Description	Action	Route Given	Frequency	Possible Side Effects	Incidence	Precautions
Methotrexate (MTX, Amethopterin)	Small yellow tablet: 2.5 mg	Interferes with action of a vitamin and thus production of DNA.	Oral	Weekly	Mouth ulcers	F	
					Nausea, vomiting	F	
					Bone marrow depression	F	
	Clear yellow liquid		IM IV IT	Variable	Loss of appetite	O	
					Hair loss	O	
					Diarrhea	R	
					Jaundice	R	
Nitrogen Mustard (Mustargen)	Clear yellowish liquid	Reacts with and damages nucleus of rapidly growing cells.	IV	Variable	Nausea, vomiting	F	Causes tissue burns if it infiltrates.
					Diarrhea	O	
					Skin rash	R	
Novantrone (Mitroxantrone Hydrochloride)	Dark blue liquid	Inhibits cell division by blocking nucleic acid production.	IV	Variable	Nausea, vomiting	F	Causes tissue burns if it infiltrates.
					Bone marrow depression	F	
					Mouth ulcers	F	Echocardiogram should be done at regular intervals.
					Blueish-green discoloration of sclera (white of eye) and urine	O	
Prednisone (Deltasone) (steroid)	White pill: 5, 20, 50 mg	Destroys lymphocytic cells.	Oral	Daily	Weigh gain, rounded face	F	Do not stop abruptly; must be tapered slowly when being discontinued.
					Mood changes	F	
					Stomach irritation	O	
					Suppression of fever and signs of inflammation and infection.	O	

Drug	Appearance	Action	Administration	Frequency	Side effects	F/O/R	Notes
Hydrocortisone (Solu-cortef) (steroid)	Clear colorless liquid		IV		Elevated blood pressure	R	
					Muscle weakness	R	
					Increased thirst and urination and increased blood sugar	R	
Procarbazine (Natulan)	White capsule: 50 mg	Inhibits protein, RNA and DNA synthesis	Oral	Variable	Nausea, vomiting	F	While taking avoid antihistamines and ripe cheese.
					Bone marrow depression	F	
					Diarrhea or constipation	O	
					Dry mouth	O	
					Fever, chills	R	
					Skin rash	R	
					Headaches, dizziness	R	
6-Thioguanine (6-TG)	Small beige tablet: 40 mg.	Inhibits production of proteins.	Oral	Daily	Bone marrow depression	F	
					Nausea, vomiting	F	
					Sore mouth	F	
Vinblastine (Velbe)	Clear liquid	Inhibits division of malignant cells.	IV	Usually once weekly or variable	Hair loss	F	May cause tissue burns if it infiltrates.
					Loss of tendon reflexes	F	
					Bone marrow depression	O	
					Constipation	O	

NOTE: For more specific information about the dosage, action, side effects, and methods of administration you should consult your child's physician.

Medication	Description	Action	Route	Frequency Given	Possible Side Effects	Incidence	Precautions
Vincristine (Oncovin)	Clear colorless liquid	Prevents division of leukemic cells.	IV	Weekly	Pains in jaw, limbs, or abdomen	O	Causes tissue burns if it infiltrates.
					Tingling in hands or feet	O	
					Loss of appetite	O	
					Leg weakness	O	
					Constipation	O	
					Hair loss	O	
VM26 (Teniposide)	Clear colorless liquid	Inhibits formation of DNA and RNA	IV	Variable	Nausea, vomiting	F	May cause tissue burns if it infiltrates.
					Bone marrow depression	F	
					Hypotension or hypertension	R	
					Fever	R	

NOTE: For more specific information about the dosage, action, side effects, and methods of administration you should consult your child's physician.

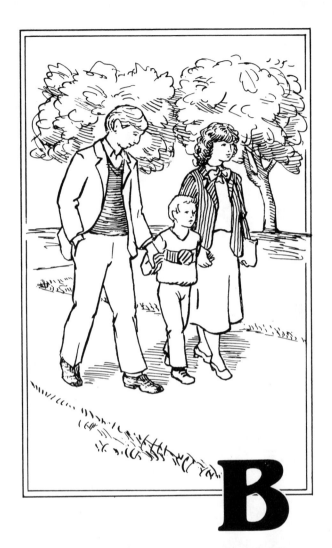

B
GLOSSARY
OF MEDICAL TERMS

Acute: Occurring suddenly; over a short period of time.

Acute Lymphocytic (Lymphatic; Lymphoblastic) Leukemia (ALL): A disorder in blood cell production in which abnormal white blood cells (lymphoblasts) multiply in the blood and bone marrow. It is the most common form of childhood leukemia.

Acute Myelogenous (Granulocytic; Myeloblastic) Leukemia (AML): The malignant cell in this disease is an immature granulocyte (myeloblast). It is more resistant to treatment than are other forms of leukemia. It is more common in people over 25 years but can occur in children.

Alopecia: Baldness; the loss of hair.

Ambulatory: Being able to walk; not confined to bed.

Anemia: A decrease in the number of circulating red blood cells (erythrocytes); a decrease in the oxygen-carrying capacity of the blood.

Anorexia: Loss of appetite.

Antibiotic: A drug used in the treatment of bacterial infections. Some antibiotics are capable of killing malignant cells and are currently used in cancer treatment.

Antibody: A substance made by lymphocytes that helps to defend the body against infections caused by bacteria and viruses.

Antigen: A foreign substance such as measles virus that stimulates the lymphocytes to produce antibodies.

Antihistamine: A medication used for treatment of allergic reactions such as hives, hay fever, etc.

Artery: A blood vessel that transports oxygen-rich blood from the heart to the tissues.

Asepsis (aseptic): Free of infection.

Aspiration: The removal of fluid or air from a body cavity by suction into a syringe.

Bacteria: A group of living one-celled organisms that are only visible through a microscope. Most are harmless; however, if the body's resistance is lowered, they can cause disease.

Barrier System: Isolation of patients from their environment to protect them from infection or to protect others.

Benign Tumor: A nonmalignant growth usually considered to be harmless.

Biopsy: A procedure in which a small piece of tissue is removed from the body by a needle or through an incision and examined under a microscope for purposes of diagnosis.

Blast Cell; Lymphoblast: The malignant cell in lymphocytic leukemia; an abnormal immature lymphocyte (white blood cell). It multiplies, causing severe crowding in the bone marrow, and thereby inhibits growth of normal cells. **Myeloblast:** The malignant cell in acute myeloblastic leukemia.

Blood Typing and Cross-Matching: Blood cells contain factors that are not the same for all people. Before a transfusion can be given, blood samples from the donor and recipient are typed and classified. The four main red blood cell types or groups are A, B, AB, and O. Once the two blood samples are typed they are then cross-matched to be sure they are compatible. This is done by placing red cells from the donor in a sample of the recipient's serum and red cells of the recipient in a sample of the donor's serum. If the blood does not agglutinate or "clump" the two bloods are compatible. Techniques for typing white blood cells and platelets are similar, but more involved.

Blood Transfusion: Procedure by which whole blood or packed red cells are given intravenously from a compatible donor.

Bone Marrow: The spongy material which fills the inner cavities of the bones. It contains the factory for producing all types of blood cells.

Bone Marrow Aspiration: The removal of a small amount of the liquid portion of the bone marrow by suction into a syringe. A sample is usually taken from one of the bones in the hip or chest.

Burkitt's Lymphoma: A rare type of lymphatic cancer.

Burns; Vincristine tissue burns: Occur when Vincristine is injected and accidentally spills outside of a vein. There may be redness, swelling, pain, and blistering as a result of damage to skin and tissue. A number of other anti-cancer drugs can cause similar burns.

Cancer: Abnormal cell growth, which can occur in any tissue of the body. It results from a change in certain cells that allows them to grow and multiply indefinitely, thereby severely interfering with the development and growth of normal tissues.

Carcinogen: A chemical or an environmental agent that can cause cancer.

Carcinoma: A malignant tumor that is composed chiefly of epithelial cells, that is, tissue that covers or lines the body surface and internal organs, for example, in the lining of the lungs and digestive tract. Such tumors are rare in children.

CAT Scan (Computerized Axial Tomography Scan): A modern x-ray technique in which a computer is used to produce a three-dimensional image of an organ or body segment.

CBC (Complete Blood Count): A test to examine the components of the blood for the purpose of diagnosis of disease or evaluation of treatment. It includes measuring hemoglobin, white cells, platelets, and a differential count.

Cell: The smallest living unit of the body. It consists of a nucleus and cytoplasm. A group of cells that come together to perform a specific function become an organ.

Central Nervous System (CNS): Consists of the brain, brainstem, and spinal cord.

Chemotherapy: Treatment using anti-cancer drugs to kill malignant cells.

Chromosomes: Rod-shaped structures found in the nucleus of a cell. They contain all the information for the cell's behavior. Chromosomes consist of thousands of genes.

Chronic: Lasting a long time.

Chronic Myelogenous Leukemia (CML): A disease similar to acute myelogenous leukemia except that it is a slowly progressive disease. It is extremely rare in children but more common in adults.

Cobalt Treatment: Radiation that uses gamma rays as a treatment for cancer limited to one area.

Colostomy: A temporary or permanent opening from the colon to the abdominal surface to allow elimination of wastes.

Coma: A state of deep and prolonged unconsciousness.

Combination Chemotherapy: Using two or more drugs at one time to treat cancer.

Congenital: Any condition that exists at birth.

Corticosteroids (Steroids): Chemical substances or hormones that destroy lymphocytes, e.g., prednisone.

Cortisone: Steroid hormone produced by the adrenal glands.

Cranial Radiation: X-ray treatment directed to the brain to prevent and destroy the growth of leukemic cells.

Cross-Matching: Test done by placing red blood cells from the donor in a sample of recipient's serum and vice versa to determine whether the two bloods do not agglutinate or "clump" together and, therefore, are compatible. This test is done prior to blood transfusion.

Culture: If an infection is suspected, samples of blood, urine, and throat secretions may be taken. In the laboratory attempts are made to grow the specific organism responsible for the infection. It may then be possible to determine which antibiotic would provide the most effective treatment.

Cyst: A malignant or benign sac filled with fluid.

Cystitis: Inflammation of the bladder that may cause burning, pain, and blood in the urine. It may result from infection or drugs such as cyclophosphamide.

Cytoplasm: The plasma surrounding the nucleus of the cell.

Cytotoxic: Destructive to cells.

Dehydration: A condition resulting from loss of water and often caused by severe diarrhea or prolonged nausea and vomiting.

Diagnosis: The process utilizing symptoms, laboratory results, and physical examination to determine the nature of a disease.

Differential Count: A test to determine the number of each of the different types of white blood cells. A small amount of blood is placed on a glass slide, and the counts are determined by microscopic examination.

Diuretic: A drug that increases the amount of water and salt eliminated from the body.

DNA (Deoxyribonucleic Acid): The substance found in the nucleus of the cell that controls the genetic characteristics of the cell.

Drug: A chemical used in the treatment, control, and/or prevention of a disease.

Edema: The accumulation of excessive fluid in the tissues. The lower legs and feet are commonly affected.

Electrolytes: Minerals such as calcium, potassium, and sodium that are needed to provide the proper environment for the cells in the body.

Emaciation: Wasting of the body.

Enzyme: A complex protein produced within an organism that controls the rate of a chemical reaction in the body. Some drugs are enzymes and can change the kind and rate of a chemical reaction in the body.

Erythrocytes (Red Blood Cells; RBC): Carry oxygen as it is breathed in through the lungs to all parts of the body. These cells are produced in the bone marrow.

Ewing's Sarcoma: A malignant tumor that arises from bones. It usually occurs in people under 20 years of age.

Excision: Surgical removal of any tissue.

Fungus: A one-celled organism that is generally harmless. Occasionally, fungi may cause serious infection in patients who have a lowered resistance.

Gamma Globulin: A protein component of the blood. Most antibodies are gamma globulins.

Gastrointestinal Tract (GI Tract): Consists of the mouth, esophagus, stomach, and intestines.

Gene: A hereditary unit made up of DNA and located in the nucleus of a cell. It controls a trait or process.

Graft Versus Host Disease (GVHD): A reaction that may develop following bone marrow transplants. Its severity will depend on how well the antigens of the recipient and donor match. Symptoms may include skin rash, blisters, diarrhea, and jaundice.

Granulocytes: One type of white blood cell that fights infection by engulfing invading bacteria. They are made in bone marrow.

Granulocytopenia: A deficiency of granulocytes in the blood.

Hemangioma: A tumor consisting mainly of dilated or newly formed blood vessels.

Hematocrit: The percentage of the blood that is made up of red blood cells.

Hematologist: A doctor specializing in the treatment of diseases of the blood.

Hematology: The branch of medicine that studies the function of blood and the blood-forming organs.

Hemoglobin: The protein in red blood cells that carries oxygen.

Hemorrhage: Loss of blood as a result of injury to blood vessels or a deficiency in platelets.

Herpes Virus: Virus that causes herpes diseases such as blisters of the skin and mouth.

Herpes Zoster: See Shingles.

Hickman Catheter: A catheter passed under the skin of the chest wall and inserted into the right chamber of the heart. See Chapter 5 for further information.

HLA (Human Leukocyte Antigens): Refers to the antigens (protein substances in the chromosomes) that determine whether tissues (i.e., bone marrow, blood, or organ) from a donor will be accepted or rejected by the recipient. These are measured on white cells.

Hodgkin's Disease: Cancer affecting the lymphatic tissues, which are important in the person's ability to fight infection. It is characterized by enlarged lymph nodes and spleen.

Hormone: Chemical substance produced by endocrine glands that helps to regulate and coordinate various body functions.

Immune reaction: The reaction of normal tissues to bacteria and viruses.

Immunity (Immune System): The blood and other body fluids contain proteins called *antibodies* that react chemically with invading organisms to destroy them.

Immunotherapy: A technique that attempts to use the body's own defenses to fight cancer. The most common method is to inject BCG (a weak bacteria) to stimulate the patient's own immune system.

Infection: Invasion of body tissues by disease-producing organisms.

Infusion: A procedure by which fluid or medication is given directly into a vein. If it is given over a period of time it is an intravenous or IV drip.

Injections: Administration of medication using a needle may be

1. Intramuscular, IM (into a muscle);
2. Intravenous, IV (into a vein);
3. Subcutaneous, SC (under the skin); or
4. Intradermal (into the skin).

Interferon: Special proteins made by cells to fight virus infections.

Intrathecal: An injection that is given directly into the spinal canal to prevent or destroy leukemia cells or to administer other medications.

Isolation: Placing patients in a special separate room to protect them from contacting any infection, especially when their immune system is weak.

Isotopic Scan: A diagnostic procedure used to examine organs. A small amount of radioactive substance is injected and then the organ is examined by x-ray or fluoroscope.

Kidney: Organ responsible for maintaining proper water and mineral balance; primary organ for the excretion of certain wastes from the body.

Laparotomy: Surgical incision through the abdominal wall to examine internal organs.

Laser: An optical instrument that emits an intense beam of hot light.

Lethargic: Drowsy, inactive.

Leukemia: Cancer of the blood that begins in the bone marrow when there is an excessive production of immature white blood cells that crowd out and inhibit the growth and development of red blood cells.

Leukocytes: White blood cells.

Leukopenia: Low white blood cell count.

Liver: An important organ that aids in digestion, produces certain blood proteins, and eliminates many waste products.

Lumbar Puncture (LP): Spinal tap. A needle is introduced into the spinal canal to remove small amounts of the cerebral spinal fluid that bathes the brain and spinal cord.

Lymph: The almost colorless liquid contained in the lymph nodes and lymphatic vessels.

Lymphatic System: All the lymphoid organs and the circulatory network of vessels that carry lymph fluid.

Lymph Nodes: Bean-shaped structures scattered along the lymphatic vessels that act as filters to collect bacteria or malignant cells. These nodes are quite small but can become very large in certain diseases.

Lymphoblast: A lymphocyte that is in an early stage of development.

Lymphocytes: A type of white blood cell formed in the lymph glands, spleen, bone marrow, and tonsils. They become active in immune reactions by producing antibodies or other defense substances.

Lymphoid Organs and Tissue: The spleen, thymus, tonsils, and the lymph nodes in the neck, armpits, groin, and other parts of the body act as a defense system by producing antibodies against foreign substances.

Lymphoma (Lymphosarcoma): A malignant tumor in the lymphatic tissue caused by the growth of abnormal lymphocytes.

Macrophages: White blood cells that attack invading germs.

Malignant: Ability to invade and actively destroy surrounding tissue.

Malignant Tumor: A cancerous growth that increases in size. Cells from this tumor can break away and be carried by the bloodstream to other parts of the body to become new tumors.

Melanoma: Dark pigmented malignant tumor usually of the skin or eye.

Meningeal Leukemia: The brain and spinal cord are covered by membranes called meninges. This leukemia occurs when these meninges are invaded by leukemic cells.

Metabolism: Refers to all the chemical changes that take place in the body and are necessary for life.

Metastasis: The spread of cancer cells and development of new tumors in another part of the body. The new growths are like the original tumor.

Microorganism: A general term for a small living organism, e.g., bacteria, fungi, and viruses.

Mitosis: Cell reproduction when one cell divides itself into two cells.

MLC (Mixed Leukocyte Culture): A test that mixes white blood cells of a donor and recipient to determine whether or not their tissue is compatible.

Modality: Refers to the type and method of treatment, e.g., surgery, chemotherapy, and radiotherapy.

Monocyte: A white blood cell that devours foreign substances and works with lymphocytes in immune reactions.

Mutation: A change in a gene occuring spontaneously or as a result of radiation or chemotherapy.

Nasal-Gastric Tube: Tube that is passed through the nose into the stomach; used for liquid feeding.

Neoplasm (Neoplastic): Any abnormal growth; usually a malignant tumor.

Neuroblastoma: Solid tumor arising from tissues of the nervous system. Often located in the abdomen.

Neurology: Study of the nervous system.

Neuroma: Tumor growing on a nerve and usually producing pain.

Neutropenia: Low neutrophil count.

Neutrophil: A white blood cell that defends the body against infection by eating bacteria, viruses, and fungi.

Non-Hodgkins Lymphoma: A tumor that develops in any lymphatic tissue of the body.

Nucleus: The dense center portion of the cell that coordinates the cell's activities.

Oncology: The study of malignant tumors.

Oncologist: A doctor who specializes in the treatment of tumors.

Organ: Several tissues grouped together to perform specific functions in the body.

Organism: A living thing.

Osteogenic Sarcoma (Osteosarcoma): A malignant tumor of the bone.

Osteoma: A tumor that is composed of bone and usually is benign.

Packed Red Blood Cells: The red blood cells remaining after the plasma has been removed from the whole blood.

Palliative: Refers to relieving the severity of the symptoms of a disease without being able to cure.

Pancytopenia: A decrease in the number of platelets and red and white blood cells.

Pathologist: A doctor who specializes in understanding disease-caused changes in body tissues.

Pathology: The study and examination of tissue to determine a diagnosis.

Petechiae: Tiny red localized hemorrhages just below the surface of the skin. In leukemia, they indicate a marked decrease in platelets and disappear when the platelet count returns to normal.

Pharmacology: The study of drugs, their absorption, distribution in the body, and excretion.

Plasma: The liquid portion of the blood containing proteins and minerals that are necessary for normal body functioning.

Platelets (thrombocytes): Particles in the blood responsible for forming clots and preventing hemorrhage.

Platelet Pack: A concentration of blood platelets given to patients with a low platelet count or with poorly functioning platelets.

Prognosis: A prediction, made by a doctor, regarding the outcome of a disease. It is based on the average outcome of treatment in similar cases.

Prosthesis: An appliance such as an artificial limb or other substitute for a missing part.

Protocol: A formal treatment plan that specifies dosages of drugs, times they are to be given, and various procedures and tests necessary during the course of treatment.

Radiation: The release of energy through x-rays or ultraviolet waves. The beam passes through objects that cannot be penetrated by visible light.

Radiation Therapy (Radiotherapy): Treatment using high energy radiation from x-ray, cobalt, or radium to destroy living cells.

Radical Surgery: An operation that removes the tumor as well as the surrounding tissues and lymph nodes.

Radioresistant: A malignant tumor that does not respond adequately to radiation.

Radiosensitive: A malignant tumor that responds to radiation, i.e., it decreases in size or is eliminated.

Red Blood Cells (Erythrocytes): Cells that carry oxygen to the organs and tissues in the body.

Relapse: The return of a disease after a period of improvement when there were few if any symptoms.

Remission: The period of time where there is a decrease in or disappearance of the symptoms of cancer.

Renal: Refers to the kidneys.

Rescue: The term used for the drug given to counteract the toxicity of another drug or drugs.

Resection: The surgical removal of any tissue.

Retinoblastoma: A rare malignant tumor that develops in the retina of the eye. It is most common in young children.

Rhabdomyosarcoma: A malignant tumor of the soft tissues of the body, usually muscle.

RNA (Ribonucleic Acid): One of the two acids found in the nucleus of the cell. It transmits the genetic information to the rest of the cell.

Sarcoma: A malignant tumor of connective tissue, cartilage, bone, fat, muscle, nerve sheath, blood vessels, or lymph tissue.

Secretion: Discharge of a substance from a cell or gland.

Sedative: A drug given to calm someone who is very anxious. May help to induce sleep.

Seizure (Convulsion; Fit): A sudden attack symptomatic of a disease such as intracranial hemorrhage. It is severe involuntary muscular contraction of the arms, legs, and body.

Septicemia: Widespread bacterial infection involving the bloodstream. Sometimes it is a result of a very low white cell count.

Shingles: Also known as herpes zoster. This infection is caused by the same virus that is responsible for chicken pox. The virus infects the nerve endings and adjacent skin resulting in painful blisters. Children who have not had chicken pox may contract it from individuals with shingles.

Spinal tap: A procedure by which a needle is inserted into the spinal canal between the vertebrae in order to withdraw spinal fluid or to inject medicine.

Spleen: An organ located in the left upper abdomen that has many lymphocytes and acts as a filter. It usually becomes enlarged in leukemia and lymphoma.

Steroids (Corticosteroids): Hormones or chemical substances that destroy lymphocytes.

Stomatitis: An inflammation of the mucous membranes of the mouth.

Subcutaneous: Under the skin.

Syndrome: A set of symptoms that usually occur together.

Systemic: Refers to the body as a whole.

Therapeutic: Refers to the treatment of a disease.

Thoracic: Refers to the thorax, which includes the chest, rib cage, and organs within the rib cage.

Thrombocytopenia: A lowered platelet count.

Thymus Gland: Located in the upper front portion of the chest behind the breastbone. It contains lymphocytes.

Tissue: A collection of cells that are similar in structure and function.

Tissue Typing: A test used to determine the HLA antigens in a given individual. This test is employed to match compatible donor and recipient in bone marrow and organ transplantation.

Tolerance: The ability to withstand treatment with a particular drug and have no ill effects.

Tomography: X-ray picture of a layer of tissue at any depth.

Toxicity (Toxic): The undesirable side effects caused by a drug, which may be mild to severe but are usually temporary.

Tumor: An abnormal swelling or growth of tissue in a localized area of the body. It can be benign or malignant. If benign and removed it does not grow again. If malignant and not completely removed it can spread in the body.

Ulcer: A deterioration of normal tissue as a result of infection, acidity, poor circulation, or malignancy.

Uric Acid: A chemical that may accumulate in the body when the kidneys do not function properly. If malignant cells are rapidly destroyed, uric acid is produced in large quantities.

Vein: A blood vessel that carries blood from the tissues to the heart and lungs.

Viruses: A group of tiny organisms, smaller than bacteria, that can produce diseases such as measles, mumps, chicken pox, and the common cold.

Vitamins: A group of chemical substances essential to maintaining normal growth and body function. They are abundant in most foods.

White Blood Cells (Leukocytes, WBC): Consist of lymphocytes, monocytes, and granulocytes that work together in bodily defense to fight infection.

White Blood Count (WBC): A test to determine the total number of leukocytes in the blood.

Wilm's Tumor: A malignant tumor that arises from the kidneys. It is most common in early childhood.

X-rays: Radiation that has the same nature as light but has an extremely short wavelength. It can be used to penetrate various thicknesses of solid to form a "picture," i.e., an image on photographic film.

Zoster Immune Globulin (ZIG): A concentrated form of zoster immune plasma.

Zoster Immune Plasma (ZIP): A plasma obtained from individuals who have had shingles. It contains antibodies against chicken pox virus. If given within 72 hours of exposure to chicken pox it can either prevent chicken pox or minimize its severity.

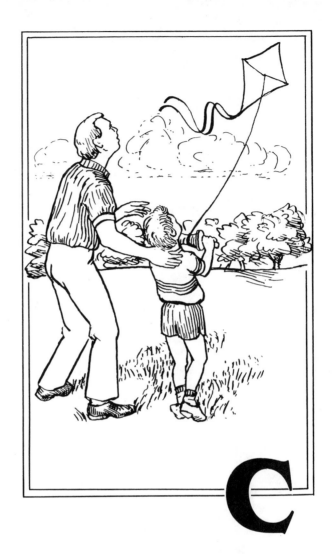

C

ADDITIONAL
READING MATERIAL

ESPECIALLY FOR PARENTS

Candlelighters National Foundation Quarterly Newsletter.

Comments: This provides information on such topics as treatment, research, and problems of living with childhood cancer. The foundation is an international organization of and for parents of children with cancer.

Source: The Candlelighters Foundation
Suite 1001
1901 Pennsylvania Ave. N.W.
Washington, D.C. 20006

Candlelighters Childhood Cancer Foundation, Canada publishes a **Newsletter** for parents.

Source: The Candlelighters Foundation, Canada
9 Church St.
Box 328
Stanstead, P.Q. JOB 3E0

Diet and Nutrition: A Resource for Parents of Children with Cancer. 1979.

Comments: This handbook was developed to serve as a source of information for parents on diet and nutrition. It also provides suggestions for coping with the nutritional problems that may occur from day to day. A poster titled "How to Build a Stronger Kid" is included as well as colorful diet sheets that can be removed and displayed for easy reference.

Source: National Cancer Institute
Office of Cancer Communications
900 Rockville Pike
Building 31, Room 10A18
Bethesda, Maryland 20205
Publication Number: 80-2038

Emotional Aspects of Childhood Cancer and Leukemia: A Handbook for Parents. Spinetta, J. J., Spinetta, P. D., Kung, F., & Schwartz, D. B. 1976.

Comments: This booklet deals with the emotional demands placed on parents and how they can cope with their feelings and those of the sick child and other family members. It also deals with suggestions on communicating with the sick child.

Source: Leukemia Society of America
San Diego Chapter
326 Broadway
San Diego, California 92101

Home Care for Dying Children: A Manual for Parents. Moldow, D. G., & Martinson, I. M. 1979.

Comments: This book describes home care and its benefits. It discusses treatments, methods for relief of pain, and information on medications and control of medical problems.

Source: University of Minnesota
School of Nursing
3313 Powell Hall
500 Essex Street, S.E.
Minneapolis, Minnesota 55455

Parent's Handbook on Leukemia. Schweers, E. W., Farnes, P., & Forman, E. N. 1977

Comments: This brochure is directed at parents of leukemic children. It provides medical and practical information to help them understand and cope with childhood leukemia. It includes information on medical procedures, medications, drug actions, and common health questions.

Source: The American Cancer Society
777 Third Avenue
New York, New York 10017
Publication Number: 4556

The Bereaved Parent. Schiff, H. S. 1977.

Comments: This book is based on personal experience as well as discussions with bereaved parents. It offers advice to parents who are facing their child's death as well as those whose child is already dead. Topics discussed include funeral arrangements and the difficulties of reestablishing family relationships and coping with delayed reactions. It is easily read, and some parents have found it to be a source of encouragement and strength.

Source: Crown Publishers, Inc.
One Park Avenue
New York, New York 10016

Paperback: Penguin Books Inc.
625 Madison Avenue
New York, New York 10022, U.S.A.

The Grief of Parents When a Child Dies. Miles, M. S. 1978.

Comments: This booklet deals with the grief of parents and siblings and how to deal with it.

Source: The Compassionate Friends, Inc.
P.O. Box 3696
Oak Brook, Illinois 60522

The Last Day of April. Roach, N. 1974.

Comments: This booklet is written by a mother who learned how to help her very young daughter adjust to her life with leukemia. It is a very personal account of how one family learned to cope and to live from day to day.

Source: The American Cancer Society
777 Third Avenue
New York, New York 10017

The Leukemic Child. Sherman, M. 1976.

Comments: In this booklet a mother who is also a journalist tells of her daughter's struggle with leukemia. She discusses the disease, her child's hospitalization, and the experiences that were encountered once her daughter returned home and then relapsed. Sections of this story deal with the way in which this child, her mother, and her two sisters coped with the emotional impact of this long-term illness and the child's death.

Source: National Cancer Institute
Office of Cancer Communications
900 Rockville Pike
Building 31, Room 10A18
Bethesda, Maryland 20205

Young People with Cancer: A Handbook for Parents. 1982

Comments: This handbook is written for parents and deals with the common questions concerning childhood cancer, medical information, and practical suggestions. It provides a general guide on what to expect during the course of the illness and how to deal with difficulties as they arise.

Source: National Cancer Institute
Office of Cancer Communications
900 Rockville Pike
Building 31, Room 10A18
Bethesda, Maryland 20205

ESPECIALLY FOR ADOLESCENTS

Candlelighters Teenage Newsletter. Quarterly.

Comments: This newsletter is written for and by adolescents who have cancer. It contains personal experiences as well as information about programs and publications that may be of interest to adolescents.

Source: Teens Newsletter
              Candlelighters Foundation
              Suite 1001
              1901 Pennsylvania Ave. N.W.
              Washington, D.C. 20006

Help Yourself: Tips for Teenagers with Cancer. 1983.

Comments: This booklet is written specifically to help teens
              and covers many topics including diagnosis,
              treatments, what to ask the doctor, how to cope
              with parents and siblings, eating problems, return
              to school and relapse.

Source: National Cancer Institute
              Office of Cancer Communications
              Building 31, Room 4B39
              Bethesda, Maryland 20205

ESPECIALLY FOR CHILDREN

Anne and the Sand Dobbies. Corburn, J. B. 1964.

Comments: This story is written from the perspective of a
              young boy. It deals with the death of his little
              sister Anne and his dog Bonnie. It is a warm and
              loving story about how death affected his family
              and is suitable for school-age children and
              parents to read.

Source: The Seabury Press
              Service Center
              Somer, Connecticut 06071

The Tenth Good Thing About Barney. Viorst, J. 1971.

Comments: This short story tells us how a little boy adjusted
              to the death of his pet cat, Barney, with the help
              and understanding of his parents. It is a story that

could be read to preschool children or read by children in grade school.

Source: Athenaeum Press
                 597 5th Avenue
                 New York, New York 10017

There Is a Rainbow Behind Every Dark Cloud. 1978.

Comments: This book is written and illustrated by children who have life-threatening illnesses. It is meant to help children deal with their fears and emphasizes living for today with a positive attitude.

Source: The Center for Attitudinal Healing
              19 Main Street
              Tiburon, California 94920

What Happened to You, Happened to Me. Kjosness, M., Rudolph, L. 1980.

Comments: This booklet, written by children who have cancer, covers several areas including hospital experiences, surgery, radiation, clinic visits, feelings, hair loss, and school activities. It is geared to school-age children with cancer.

Source: Children's Orthopedic Hospital and Medical Center
              Division of Pediatric Hematology/Oncology
              4800 Sand Point Way, P.E.
              P.O. Box C5371
              Seattle, Washington 98105

When Your Brother or Sister Has Cancer. Rudolph, L. 1980.

Comments: This booklet has been written for children ranging from grade school age to early adolescence. It helps brothers and sisters to understand their reactions and feelings when their sibling has cancer.

Source: Children's Orthopedic Hospital and Medical Center

Division of Pediatric Hematology/Oncology
4800 Sand Point Way, P.E.
P.O. Box C5371
Seattle, Washington 98105

You and Leukemia: A Day at a Time. Baker, L. 1976.

Comments: This handbook is written for children who have
leukemia. It is filled with explanations and il-
lustrations about leukemia, what it does, and how
to treat it.

Source: W. B. Saunders Company
West Washington Square
Philadelphia, Pennsylvania 19105

ESPECIALLY FOR TEACHERS

Cancer in the Classroom: How Do You Cope? Klopovich, P.,
Rosen, D., Cairns, N., & Moore, R.

Comments: This pamphlet covers several important areas and is
a good guide for teachers. Topics discussed include
an explanation about cancer, treatment, and side
effects. Problems that may affect school behavior
and attendance as well as special concerns for high
school students are covered. There is also a section
that discusses what the teacher should expect and
how to handle issues that may arise when a child
dies.

Source: Mid-American Cancer Center
University of Kansas Medical Center
National Cancer Institute
Bethesda, Maryland 20205

Students with Cancer: A Resource for the Educator. 1980

Comments: This booklet provides general information regarding cancer, treatment, and side effects. It provides guidelines for the teacher regarding school

reentry and dealing with parents and classmates. It also discusses terminal illness and provides information on additional reading material for teachers and young people.

Source: U.S. Department of Health and Human Services
Public Health Service
National Institutes of Health
National Cancer Institute
Bethesda, Maryland 20205
Publication Number: 80-2086

NEW BOOKS

Childhood Cancer and the Family: Meeting the Challenge of Stress and Support. Chesler, M.A. & Barbarin, O. 1987.

Comments: This book focusses on the psychosocial aspects of childhood cancer and integrates scientific data with the experiences of families.

Source: Brunner/Mazel Publishers
19 Union Square
New York, New York 1003, U.S.A.

Suffer the Little Children. Demers, J. 1986.

Comments: A physician offers a touching and personal account of his work with children with cancer and their families.

Source: Eden Press
4626 St. Catherine St. W.
Montreal, P.Q., Canada H3Z 1S3

My Book for Kids with Cansur. Gaes, J. 1987.

Comments: An 8 year old boy describes his thoughts and feelings. It is vividly illustrated and written for young children.

Source: Melius & Peterson Publishing, Inc.
Rm. 524, 202 S. Main St.
P.O. Box 925, Aberdeen, South Dakota 57401

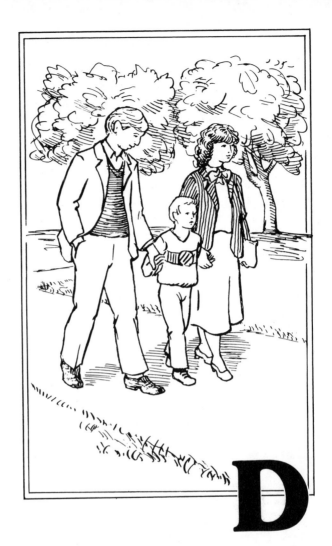

D

BIBLIOGRAPHY

Adams, D. W. *Childhood malignancy: The psychosocial care of the child and his family.* Springfield IL: Charles C Thomas, 1979.

Adams, D. W. *The psychosocial care of the child and his family in childhood cancer: An annototated bibliography.* Hamilton, Ontario: McMaster University Medical Centre, 1979.

Aradine, C. R. Books for children about death. *Pediatrics,* 1976, 57(3), 372–378.

Baker, I. S., Roland, C. G, & Gilchrist, G. S. *You and leukemia: A day at a time.* Rochester MN: Mayo Comprehensive Cancer Center, 1976. Also published by W. B. Saunders Co., Philadelphia, 1978.

Bluebond-Langner, M. *The private worlds of dying children.* Princeton NJ: Princeton University Press, 1978.

Blumberg, B., Flaherty, M., & Lewis, J. *Coping with cancer.* Bethesda MD: U.S. Dept. of Health and Human Services, 1980.

Cain, A. C., & Cain, B. S. "On Replacing a Child." *American Journal of the Academy of Child Psychiatry,* 1964, 3, 444.

Cairns, N. U., Clark, G. M., Smith, S. D., & Lansky, S. B. Adaptation of siblings to childhood malignancy. *Journal of Pediatrics,* 1979, 95, 484–487.

Cantor, R. C. *And a time to live: Toward emotional well being during the crisis of cancer.* New York: Harper & Row, 1978.

Comerford, B. Parental anticipatory grief and guidelines for caregivers. In B. Schoenberg et al. (Eds.), *Anticipatory grief.* New York: Columbia University Press, 1974.

Deliman, T., & Smolowe, J. S. *Holistic medicine: Harmony of body, mind, spirit.* Reston VA; Reston Publishing Co., 1982.

Goggin, E. L., Lansky, S. B., & Hassanein, K. Psychological reactions of children with malignancies. *Journal of Child Psychiatry,* 1976, 15, 314–325.

Grollman, E. A. (Ed.). *Explaining death to children.* Boston: Beacon Press, 1967.

Grollman, E. A. (Ed.). *Talking about death: A dialogue between parent and child.* Boston: Beacon Press, 1971.

Haghbin, M., Tan, C. C., Clarkson, B. D., Mike, V., Burchenal, J., & Murphy, M. L. Intensive chemotherapy in children with acute lymphoblastic leukemia (L2 protocol). *Cancer, 1974, 33(6),* 1491–1498.

Hofmann, A. D., Becker, R. D., & Gabriel, H. P. *The hospitalized adolescent: A guide to managing the ill and injured youth.* New York: The Free Press, 1976.

Holmes, G. E., & Holmes, F. F. Pregnancy outcome of patients treated for Hodgkin's disease: A controlled study. *Cancer, 1978, 41,* 1317–1322.

Holmes, H. A., & Holmes, F. F. After ten years, what are the handicaps and life styles of children treated for cancer? *Clinical Pediatrics, 1975, 14,* 819–823.

Howell, D. A. A child dies. *Journal of Pediatric Surgery, 1966, 1,* 2–7.

Hutchison, G. B. Late neoplastic changes following medical irradiation. *Radiology, 1972, 105,* 645–652.

Hutter, R. V., Shipkey, F. H., Tan, C. T., Murphy, M. L., & Chowdhury, M. Hepatic fibrosis in children with acute leukemia: A complication of therapy. *Cancer, 1960, 13,* 288–307.

Jackson, E. N. *Telling a child about death.* New York: Hawthorn Books, 1965.

Jaffe, N. Non-oncogenic sequelae of cancer chemotherapy. *Radiology, 1975, 114,* 167–173.

Jaffe, N. The cost of therapy. In J. Van Eys (Ed.), *The normally sick child.* Baltimore: University Park Press, 1979.

Jenkin, D., Freedman, M., McClure, P., Peters, V., Saunders, F., & Sonley, M. Hodgkin's disease in children: Treatment with low dose radiation and MOPP without staging laparotomy; A preliminary report. *Cancer, 1979, 44,* 80–86.

Johnson, F. L., Thomas, E. D., Clark, B. S., Chard, R. L., Hartmann, J. R., & Storb, R. A comparison of marrow transplantation with chemotherapy for children with acute lymphocytic leukemia in second or subsequent remission. *New England Journal of Medicine, 1981, 305,* 846–851.

Kaplan, D. M., Grobstein, R., & Smith, A. Predicting the impact of severe illness in families. *Health and Social Work, 1976, 1(3),* 72–82. 1976, Also see *Med World News,* April 6, 1973, p. 23.

Klinzing, D. R., & Klinzing, D. G. *The hospitalized child: Communication techniques for health personnel.* Englewood Cliffs NJ: Prentice-Hall, 1977.

Koocher, G. P., & O'Malley, J. E. *The Damocles syndrome.* New York: McGraw-Hill, 1981.

Knudson, A. G. Genetics and etiology of childhood cancer. *Pediatric Research,* 1976, *10,*513–517.

Kubler-Ross, E. *Questions and answers on death and dying.* New York: Macmillan, 1974.

Li, F. P. Follow-up of survivors of childhood cancer. *Cancer,* 1977, *39,* 1776–1778.

Li, F. P. Second malignant tumors after cancer in childhood. *Cancer,* 1977, *40,* 1899–1902.

Li, F. P., Cassady, J. R. & Jaffe,N. Risk of second tumors in survivors of childhood cancer. *Cancer,* 1975, *35,* 1230-1235.

Li, F. P., Fine, W., Jaffe, N., Holmes, G. E., & Holmes, F. F. Offspring of patients treated for cancer in childhood. *Journal of the National Cancer Institute,* 1979, *62,* 1193–1197.

Li, F. P., & Jaffe, N. Progeny of childhood cancer survivors. *Lancet,* 1974, *2* (7882), 707–709.

Li, F. P., Myers, M. H., Heise, H. W., & Jaffe, N. The course of five-year survivors of cancer in childhood. *Journal of Pediatrics,* 1978, *93,* 185-187.

Lonetto, R. *Children's conceptions of death.* New York: Springer Publishing Company, 1980.

Marshall, J. G., & Marshall, V. W. The treatment of death in children's books. *Omega,* 1971, *2,* 36–44.

Mayfield, J. K., Riseborough, E. J., & Jaffe, N. Irradiation effect on the axial skeleton following treatment for neuroblastoma. *Proceedings: American Society of Clinical Oncology/American Academy of Cancer Research,* 1977, *18,* 279.

McCollum, A. T. *Coping with prolonged health impairment in your child.* Boston: Little, Brown & Company, 1975.

Moldow, D. G. & Martinson, I. *Home care: A manual for parents.* Minneapolis: University of Minnesota, 1979.

Moody, R. A., Jr. *Life after life.* New York: Bantam Books, 1975.

Mulholland, C. *I'll dance with the rainbows.* Glasgow: Partick Press, 1973.

Parkes, C. M. *Bereavement.* London: Tavistock Publications, 1972.

Schiefelbein, S. Children and cancer: New hope for survival. *The Saturday Review,* April 14, 1979, 11–16.

Schiff, H. S. *The bereaved parent.* New York: Crown Publishers, 1977.

Schweers, E., Farnes, P., & Forman, E. *Parents' handbook on leukemia* (Rev. ed.). Rhode Island Hospital, Providence, Rhode Island: American Cancer Society, 1977.

Share, L. Family communication in the crisis of a child's fatal illness: A literature review and analysis. *Omega*, 1972, *3*, 187–201.

Sherman, M. *The leukemic child.* Washington, DC: U.S. Department of Health and Human Services, 1976.

Simonton, P. C., & Simonton, S.: *Getting well again: A self-guide to overcoming cancer.* New York: Bantam Books, 1980.

Simpson, M. *The facts of death.* Englewood Cliffs NJ: Prentice-Hall, 1979.

Spinetta, J. J. The dying child's awareness of death: A review. *Psychological Bulletin*, 1974, *81*, 256-260.

Spinetta, J. J. Adjustment in children with cancer. *Journal of Pediatric Psychology*, 1977, *2*, 49–51.

Spinetta, J. J., & Deasey Spinetta, P. *Living with Childhood Cancer.* St. Louis MO: C. V. Mosby, 1981.

Spinetta, J. J. & Maloney, L. J. Death anxiety in the outpatient leukemic child. *Pediatrics*, 1975, *65*, 1034–1037.

Spinetta, J. J., Rigler, D. & Karon, M. Anxiety in the dying child. *Pediatrics*, 1973, *52*, 841–845.

Spinetta, J. J., Rigler, D. & Karon, M. Personal space as measure of a dying child's sense of isolation. *Journal of Consulting and Clinical Psychology*, 1974, *42*, 751–756.

Spinetta, J. J., Spinetta, P. D., Kung, F., & Schwartz, D. B. *Emotional aspects of childhood cancer and leukemia: A handbook for parents.* San Diego: Leukemia Society of America, 1976.

Van Eys, J. *The truly cured child.* Baltimore: University Park Press, 1977.

Wolfe, A. *Helping your child to understand death.* New York: Child Study Association of America, 1958.

ADDITIONAL READING

Clavell, L. et al. Four Agent Induction and Intensive Asparaginase Therapy for Treatment of Childhood Acute Lymphocytic Leukemia. *New England Journal of Medicine*, 1986, 11, 657-663.

Corr, C.A. & McNeil, J.N. (Eds.) *Adolescence and Death.* New York: Springer, 1986.

Knapp, R.J. *Beyond Endurance.* New York: Schocken Books, 1986.

Rando, T. (Ed.) *Parental Loss of a Child.* Champaign, Illinois: Research Press, 1986.

Rosen, H. *Unspoken Grief: Coping with Childhood Sibling Loss.* Lexington, Mass.: D.C. Heath, 1986.

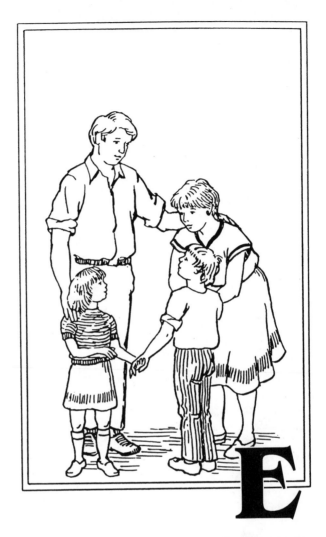

E

ADDITIONAL
SUPPORT
AND INFORMATION
FOR FAMILIES

HELP FOR PARENTS

Parent Support Groups

In many centers, parents' groups provide on-going support and opportunities to share feelings, concerns and information. They may also take part in fund raising for cancer research and participate in activities that encourage changes within hospitals and governments to meet the needs of children with cancer and their families. These groups often provide support for bereaved parents.

Some groups are formed within hospitals and many are affiliated with the Candlelighters Foundations,* local Cancer Societies and The Compassionate Friends, Inc.** Clinic staff can help you to contact the parents' group in your area.

Accommodation

Ronald McDonald Houses are usually located near Cancer Treatment Centers and provide low cost accommodation, as well as support, to parents and their families who live at a distance but must remain near the center. Some hospitals have other types of subsidized lodging. Clinic staff can help you make arrangements if accommodation is available.

Financial Concerns

In some countries, tax deductions may be provided when parents encounter uninsured medical, travel or other illness-related expenses. It is important to obtain information concerning such deductions early in your child's illness. You may direct your inquiries to the Taxation Information Center in your area.

* address p. 279
** address p. 281

As an employee, it is important to be aware of all the benefits available to you, for example, time off work for your child's hospital visits. When your child becomes ill, you may wish to contact your employer's personnel office or your local union representative.

In some states and provinces, special allowances are provided by the government for children who are very ill or disabled. The hospital social worker or clinic nurse may be able to provide you with information concerning application for appropriate benefits.

HELP FOR CHILDREN WITH CANCER

Hospital Groups

Many hospitals and treatment centers have developed special groups for children and adolescents with cancer. On-going support as well as opportunities to share feelings and concerns in a non-threatening environment help these children cope with living with cancer. If such a program is available in your area, clinic staff can help your child decide if he or she would like to participate.

Camps

Summer, winter and weekend camps provide opportunities for children to enjoy outdoor activities, gain support and form friendships with other children facing similar problems. These camps are equipped with medical facilities and doctors and nurses are available to administer chemotherapy and handle emergencies. Parents are sometimes invited to join in the fun.

Information about camps in your area can be obtained from clinic staff or from local or national branches of the Candlelighters Foundation* or the Cancer Society.

* address p. 279

HELP FOR SIBLINGS

Hospital Groups

More clinics are developing special groups for brothers and sisters of children with cancer. They provide support, opportunities to express difficult feelings and share information about cancer, the hospital and treatments. If a program for siblings is available in your area, clinic staff can help your healthy children decide if they would like to join.

Camps

In addition to camps for children with cancer, programs are offered for siblings to join their brother or sister or to go on their own to a camp just for siblings. Such programs offer unique opportunities to enjoy the outdoors, share their experiences and develop friendships. Information can be obtained from clinic staff, the Candlelighters Foundation* or the Cancer Society.

Bereavement Groups

In some areas, bereavement groups are available for children and adolescents. They provide professional guidance in a small group that encourages children to share their difficult feelings and work through their loss. If such a group is available in your area, information can be obtained from clinic staff, the Cancer Society, Candlelighters Foundation* or The Compassionate Friends, Inc.**

* address p. 279
** address p. 281

INDEX

For additional medical terms and definitions see Glossary, pages 263-275.

299

ORDER FORM

Please send me:

_____ copies of **COPING WITH CHILDHOOD CANCER: WHERE DO WE GO FROM HERE?** @ $21.95 per copy.

Shipping and handling: $1.75 first copy, $0.75 each additional copy.

All orders outside Canada: $19.95 U.S. funds.

Enclosed please find my cheque or money order payable to **KINBRIDGE PUBLICATIONS**

for the following amount $ _____

NAME: _____

ADDRESS: _____

CITY: _____ PROVINCE/STATE _____

POSTAL/ZIP CODE _____ COUNTRY _____

MAIL TO: KINBRIDGE PUBLICATIONS
P.O. BOX 5035, STATION E
HAMILTON, ONTARIO L8S 4K9
CANADA

Your help in making this book known is appreciated

POLICIES:

Price subject to change without notice.
All sales final.
Discounts for group and hospital orders.
Allow 6 to 8 weeks for delivery.

ORDER FORM

ORDER FORM

Please send me:

_____ copies of **COPING WITH CHILDHOOD CANCER: WHERE DO WE GO FROM HERE?** @ $21.95 per copy.

Shipping and handling: $1.75 first copy, $0.75 each additional copy.

All orders outside Canada: $19.95 U.S. funds.

Enclosed please find my cheque or money order payable to **KINBRIDGE PUBLICATIONS**
for the following amount $ _____

NAME:_____

ADDRESS:_____

CITY:_____ PROVINCE/STATE _____

POSTAL/ZIP CODE_____ COUNTRY _____

MAIL TO: KINBRIDGE PUBLICATIONS
P.O. BOX 5035, STATION E
HAMILTON, ONTARIO L8S 4K9
CANADA

Your help in making this book known is appreciated

POLICIES:

Price subject to change without notice.
All sales final.
Discounts for group and hospital orders.
Allow 6 to 8 weeks for delivery.

ORDER FORM

ORDER FORM

Please send me:

_____ copies of **COPING WITH CHILDHOOD CANCER: WHERE DO WE GO FROM HERE?** @ $21.95 per copy.

Shipping and handling: $1.75 first copy, $0.75 each additional copy.

All orders outside Canada: $19.95 U.S. funds.

Enclosed please find my cheque or money order payable to **KINBRIDGE PUBLICATIONS**

for the following amount $ _____

NAME: _____

ADDRESS: _____

CITY: _____ PROVINCE/STATE _____

POSTAL/ZIP CODE _____ COUNTRY _____

MAIL TO: KINBRIDGE PUBLICATIONS
P.O. BOX 5035, STATION E
HAMILTON, ONTARIO L8S 4K9
CANADA

Your help in making this book known is appreciated

POLICIES:

Price subject to change without notice.
All sales final.
Discounts for group and hospital orders.
Allow 6 to 8 weeks for delivery.

ORDER FORM